MERRILL'S
POCKET GUIDE
to RADIOGRAPHY

MERRILL'S

POCKET GUIDE
to RADIOGRAPHY

Fourteenth Edition

Bruce W. Long
MS, RT(R)(CV), FASRT, FAEIRS

Director and Associate Professor
Radiologic and Imaging Sciences
  Programs
Indiana University School of Medicine
Indianapolis, Indiana

Jeannean Hall Rollins
MRC, BSRT(R)(CV)

Associate Professor
Medical Imaging and Radiation
  Sciences Department
Arkansas State University
Jonesboro, Arkansas

Barbara J. Smith
MS, RT(R)(QM), FASRT, FAEIRS

Instructor, Radiologic Technology
Medical Imaging Department
Portland Community College
Portland, Oregon

ELSEVIER

ELSEVIER

3251 Riverport Lane
St. Louis, Missouri 63043

MERRILL'S POCKET GUIDE TO RADIOGRAPHY   ISBN: 978-0-323-59703-6

Copyright © 2019 Elsevier, Inc. All rights reserved.
Previous editions copyrighted *2016, 2012, 2007, 2003, 1999 and 1995.*

No part of this publication may be reproduced or transmitted in any form or by
any means, electronic or mechanical, including photocopying, recording, or any
information storage and retrieval system, without permission in writing from the
publisher. Details on how to seek permission, further information about the Publisher's
permissions policies and our arrangements with organizations such as the Copyright
Clearance Center and the Copyright Licensing Agency, can be found at our website:
www.elsevier.com/permissions.

This book and the individual contributions contained in it are protected under copyright
by the Publisher (other than as may be noted herein).

Notices

Practitioners and researchers must always rely on their own experience and knowledge
in evaluating and using any information, methods, compounds or experiments described
herein. Because of rapid advances in the medical sciences, in particular, independent
verifi cation of diagnoses and drug dosages should be made. To the fullest extent
of the law, no responsibility is assumed by Elsevier, authors, editors or contributors
for any injury and/or damage to persons or property as a matter of products liability,
negligence or otherwise, or from any use or operation of any methods, products,
instructions, or ideas contained in the material herein.

Library of Congress Control Number: 2018959059

Content Strategist: Sonya Seigafuse
Content Development Manager: Lisa Newton
Content Development Specialist: Betsy McCormac
Publishing Services Manager: Shereen Jameel
Project Manager: Nadhiya Sekar
Designer: Brian Salisbury

Printed in United States of America

Last digit is the print number: 9   8   7   6   5   4   3   2   1

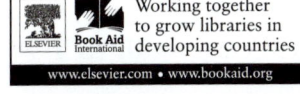

Working together
to grow libraries in
developing countries

www.elsevier.com • www.bookaid.org

Merrill's Pocket Guide to Radiography concisely presents essential positioning information for the most frequently requested projections in a format designed for quick reference. This edition offers step-by-step explanations of methods to position the patient and body part for more than 150 of the most commonly requested radiography projections, including mobile.

Its format makes the *Pocket Guide* particularly easy to use, with each projection presented in a broadside, two-page spread. Each projection presentation includes the following information:
- Patient position
- Part position
- Central ray angulation
- Collimation
- kVp
- Photograph of properly positioned patient
- Footnote that references information in the 14th edition of *Merrill's Atlas*
- Exposure technique chart with space for writing manual and automatic exposure control (AEC) technical factors (a sample of this chart with instructions for completion may be found on the next page after the contents)
- Competency check-off for students—blank lines are present on each projection page for the instructor to sign and date after the student has demonstrated competency for that projection
- Specific collimation sizing for use with DR systems

Features designed to enhance the utility of the *Pocket Guide* include section dividers with tabs, which make finding the beginning of each section easier, and abbreviations and external landmarks printed on the inside of the covers for quick reference.

Introduction

Preface

The *Pocket Guide* has grown in use by students and radiographers since it was first published in 1989. Many new features have been added since that time. Recent additions have included digital radiography notations, digital collimation, charts for automatic exposure control (AEC) techniques, and compensating filter notations. The *Pocket Guide* can also be used to keep a record of student competencies. This edition is full-featured, with the inclusion of an optimal radiograph for each projection.

We are encouraged that the *Pocket Guide* is the most widely used guide among students. Users are encouraged to send us suggestions for improvements. We sincerely hope you will find this edition of the *Pocket Guide* useful in your everyday work as a radiographer.

Recognition of Previous Author

The authors thank Philip W. Ballinger, PhD, RT(R), FAEIRS, FASRT, the second author of *Merrill's Atlas*, for his work on the previous five editions of this *Pocket Guide*. Dr. Ballinger developed the concept of providing students with a pocket-sized "guide" containing the essential projections of the *Atlas* in 1987. Eugene D. Frank, MA, RT(R), FASRT, FAEIRS, the third author of the *Atlas* continued to improve the *Pocket Guide* during his years leading the author team. The *Pocket Guide* has proven to be a very popular and valuable resource for radiography students since its inception.

Bruce W. Long
blong@iupui.edu

Jeannean Hall Rollins
jrollins@astate.edu

Barbara J. Smith
bsmith@pcc.edu

Contents

Upper Extremity, 1

Lower Extremity, 71

Vertebral Column, 137

Thorax, 185

Abdomen, 215

Cranium, 271

Mobile Radiography, 319

APPENDICES
SID Conversion, 342
Grid Conversion Factors, 344
Notes, 347

How to Use the Technical Factors Chart

Part Thickness
A given technique always depends on the thickness of the body part.

mA
Set an mA that enables use of the small focal spot whenever possible.

kVp
The kVp should be set to penetrate the body part, ensure optimum image quality at the lowest dose.

Time
Time always varies with part thickness and respiration considerations.

CR, DR Exposure Indicator
Indicate the exposure index, S number, or REX number.

HF, 1Ø, or 3Ø
Always indicate the generator phase. A 3Ø 12p requires 50% less mAs than a 1Ø 2p. A 1Ø 2p requires 50% more mAs than a 3Ø 12p.*

Manual Factors									
Part Thickness (cm)	mA	kVp	Time	mAs	SID	Image Receptor Size	CR, DR Exposure Indicator	Grid	HF 1Ø, or 3Ø
21	200	80	0.30	60	40"	14 × 17	400	12:1	3Ø 12p

AEC Factors									
Part Thickness (cm)	mA	kVp	AEC Detector	Density Comp.	SID	IR Size	CR, DR Exposure Indicator	Grid	HF 1Ø or 3Ø
21	200	80		0	48"	14 × 17	400	12:1	3Ø 12p

Detectors
Shade in the detector or detectors used for the body part.

Density Compensation
Indicate if a +1 or +2 or a −1 or −2 compensation is required for the exposure.

Digital Indicator
The exposure index for the system in use and projection should be entered here.

Example of the way technical factors would be entered for an AP projection of the pelvis in two different rooms. One room uses AEC, and the other uses manual technical factors.

See imaging textbooks for other 1Ø and 3Ø variables.

Second Through Fifth Digits:
PA, 2
Lateral, 4
PA oblique (lateral rotation), 6

First Digit (Thumb):
AP, 8
Lateral, 10
PA oblique, 12

Hand:
PA, 14
PA oblique (lateral rotation), 16
Lateral, 18

Wrist:
PA, 20
Lateral, 22
PA oblique (lateral rotation), 24
PA: ulnar deviation, 26
PA axial; STECHER METHOD, 28

Carpal Canal:
Tangential; GAYNOR-HART METHOD, 30

Forearm:
AP, 32
Lateral, 34

Elbow:
AP, 36
Lateral, 38
AP oblique (medial rotation), 40
AP oblique (lateral rotation), 42
AP partial flexion, 44

Humerus:
AP, 46
Lateral, 48

Proximal Humerus/Shoulder:
Transthoracic lateral; LAWRENCE METHOD, 50

Shoulder:
AP, 52

Shoulder Joint:
AP oblique; GRASHEY METHOD, 54

Shoulder:
Inferosuperior axial; LAWRENCE METHOD, 56
Scapular Y: PA oblique, 58

Acromioclavicular Articulations:
AP; PEARSON METHOD, 60

Clavicle:
AP, 62
AP axial, 64

Scapula:
AP, 66
Lateral, 68

Upper Extremity

Second Through Fifth Digits
PA

Patient Position
- Seat patient at end of radiographic table.

Part Position
- Place extended digit of interest with palmar surface of hand down on the IR.
- Separate digits slightly, and center the digit under examination to the center of the IR.
- Shield gonads.

Central Ray
- Perpendicular, entering PIP joint of digit being examined

Collimation:
1 inch (2.5 cm) all sides of digit, including 1 inch (2.5 cm) proximal to MCP joint. Place side marker in the collimated exposure field.

kVp: 63

Reference: 14th edition ATLAS p. 1:154.

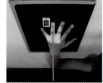
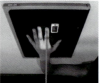
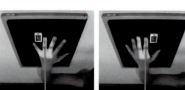

Manual Factors									
Part Thickness (cm)	mA	kVp	Time	mAs	SID	Image Receptor Size	CR, DR Exposure Indicator	Grid	HF, 1Ø or 3Ø

Notes: _____

Competency: _____/___/___

Instructor: _____

Upper Extremity

Second Through Fifth Digits
Lateral

Patient Position
• Seat patient at end of radiographic table.

Part Position
• Demonstrate position for patient. Ask patient to extend digit of interest and to close rest of digits into a fist.
• Adjust digit of interest parallel to IR plane.
• Rest digit on lateral or medial surface as needed to obtain smallest possible OID.
• Immobilize extended digit. (Use cotton swab or tape.)
• Shield gonads.

Central Ray
• Perpendicular, entering PIP joint

Collimation:
1 inch (2.5 cm) all sides of digit, including 1 inch (2.5 cm) proximal to MCP joint. Place side marker in the collimated exposure field.

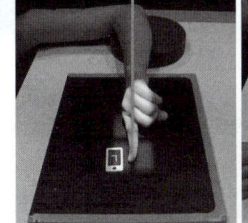
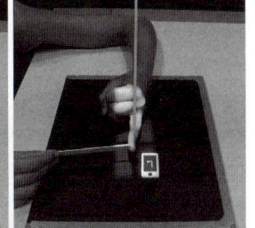

kVp: 63

Reference: 14th edition ATLAS p. 1:156.

Manual Factors									
Part Thickness (cm)	mA	kVp	Time	mAs	SID	Image Receptor Size	CR, DR Exposure Indicator	Grid	HF, 1Ø or 3Ø

Notes: _____

Competency: ___/___/___

Instructor: _____

Upper Extremity

Second Through Fifth Digits
PA oblique (lateral rotation)

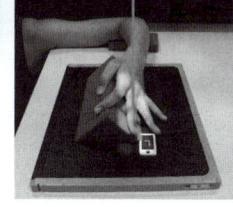
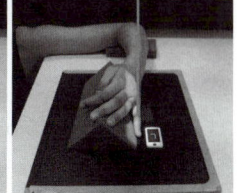

Patient Position
• Seat patient at end of radiographic table.

Part Position
• Place patient's hand in lateral position, ulnar side down and centered to IR area.
• Rotate palm 45 degrees toward IR until digits are resting on sponge support.
• Immobilize separated digits.
• Shield gonads.

Central Ray
• Perpendicular, entering PIP joint

Collimation:
1 inch (2.5 cm) on all sides of digit, including 1 inch (2.5 cm) proximal to MCP joint. Place side marker in the collimated exposure field.

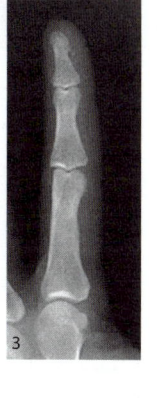

kVp: 63

Reference: 14th edition ATLAS p. 1:158.

Manual Factors									
Part Thickness (cm)	mA	kVp	Time	mAs	SID	Image Receptor Size	CR, DR Exposure Indicator	Grid	HF, 1Ø or 3Ø

Notes: _____ Competency: _____/____/____

Instructor: _____

Upper Extremity

First Digit (Thumb)
AP

Patient Position
• Seat patient at end of radiographic table.

Part Position
• Place affected hand in extreme internal rotation, with first digit centered to IR area.
• Adjust position of hand to ensure true AP projection of first digit.
• Extend and secure digits two through five to eliminate superimposition over first digit.
• Shield gonads.

Central ray
• Perpendicular, entering MCP joint of first digit

Collimation:
1 inch (2.5 cm) on all sides of digit, including 1 inch (2.5 cm) proximal to CMC joint. Place side marker in the collimated exposure field.

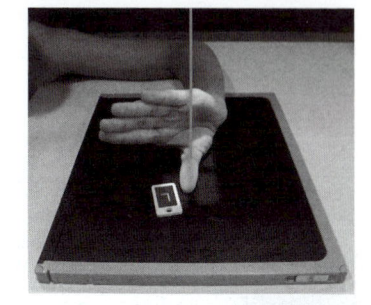

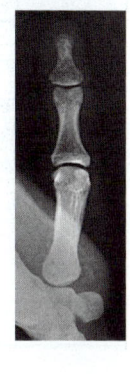

kVp: 63

Reference: 14th edition ATLAS p. 1:160.

Manual Factors									
Part Thickness (cm)	mA	kVp	Time	mAs	SID	Image Receptor Size	CR, DR Exposure Indicator	Grid	HF, 1Ø or 3Ø

Notes: _____ Competency: ____/____/____

_____ Instructor: _____

Upper Extremity

First Digit (Thumb)
Lateral

Patient Position
• Seat patient at end of radiographic table.

Part Position
• Have patient rest palmar surface of hand on IR.
• Adjust arching of hand until true lateral position of first digit is achieved.
• Shield gonads.

Central Ray
• Perpendicular, entering MCP joint of first digit

Collimation:
1 inch (2.5 cm) on all sides of digit, including 1 inch (2.5 cm) proximal to CMC joint. Place side marker in the collimated exposure field.

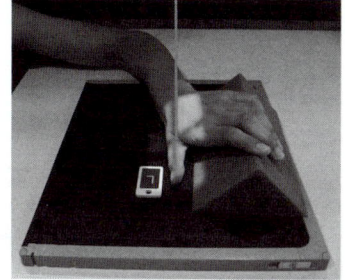
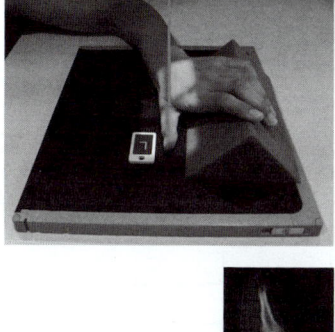

kVp: 63

Reference: 14th edition ATLAS p. 1:160.

Manual Factors									
Part Thickness (cm)	mA	kVp	Time	mAs	SID	Image Receptor Size	CR, DR Exposure Indicator	Grid	HF, 1Ø or 3Ø

Notes: _____ Competency: ____/____/____

_____ Instructor: _____

Upper Extremity

First Digit (Thumb)
PA oblique

Patient Position
• Seat patient at end of radiographic table.

Part Position
• Abduct first digit.
• Place palmar surface of hand firmly against IR, and adjust first digit to oblique position.
• Shield gonads.

Central Ray
• Perpendicular, entering MCP joint of first digit

Collimation:
1 inch (2.5 cm) on all sides of digit, including 1 inch (2.5 cm) proximal to CMC joint. Place side marker in the collimated exposure field.

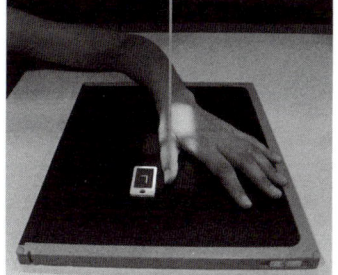

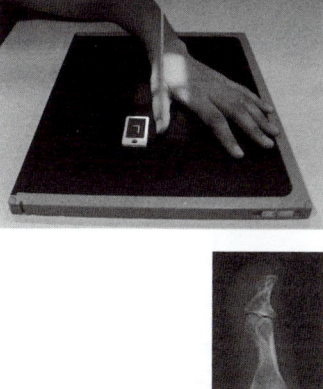

kVp: 63　　　　　　　　　*Reference: 14th edition ATLAS p. 1:160.*

Manual Factors									
Part Thickness (cm)	mA	kVp	Time	mAs	SID	Image Receptor Size	CR, DR Exposure Indicator	Grid	HF, 1Ø or 3Ø

Notes: _____ Competency: _____/____/____

_____ Instructor: _____

Upper Extremity

Hand
PA

Patient Position
- Seat patient at end of radiographic table.

Part Position
- Rest forearm on table with palmar surface of hand against IR.
- Spread digits slightly.
- Shield gonads.

Central Ray
- Perpendicular to third MCP joint

Collimation:
1 inch (2.5 cm) all sides of hand including 1 inch (2.5 cm) proximal to ulnar styloid. Place side marker in the collimated exposure field.

kVp: 66

Reference: 14th edition ATLAS p. 1:168.

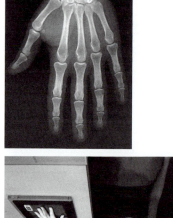
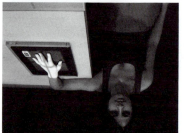

Manual Factors										
Part Thickness (cm)	mA	kVp	Time	mAs	SID	Image Receptor Size	CR, DR Exposure Indicator	Grid	HF, 1Ø or 3Ø

Notes: _____

Competency: _____/____/____

Instructor: _____

Upper Extremity

Hand
PA oblique (lateral rotation)

Patient Position
• Seat patient at end of radiographic table.

Part Position
• Rest forearm on table with palmar surface of hand against IR.
• Rotate hand laterally (externally), and place digits on 45-degree radiolucent support to show interphalangeal joints. Adjust digits parallel with IR.
• When metacarpals are area of primary interest, rotate hand laterally so that fingertips touch IR.
• Shield gonads.

Central Ray
• Perpendicular to third MCP joint

Collimation:
1 inch (2.5 cm) on all sides of hand including 1 inch (2.5 cm) proximal to ulnar styloid. Place side marker in the collimated exposure field.

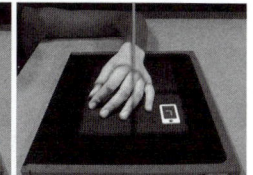
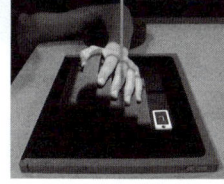
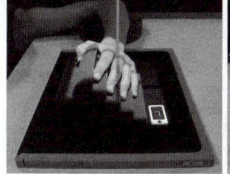

kVp: 66

Reference: 14th edition ATLAS p. 1:170.

Manual Factors									
Part Thickness (cm)	mA	kVp	Time	mAs	SID	Image Receptor Size	CR, DR Exposure Indicator	Grid	HF, 1Ø or 3Ø

Notes: _____ Competency: _____/___/___

_____ Instructor: _____

Upper Extremity

Hand
Lateral

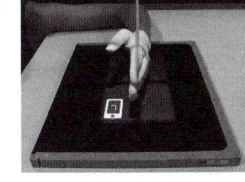

Patient Position
• Seat patient at end of radiographic table.

Part Position
• Rest ulnar surface of forearm on table with hand in true lateral position.
• Extend digits with first digit (thumb) placed at right angles to palm of hand. As an option, have patient "fan" fingers and place on positioning sponge to reduce superimposition of phalanges (as illustrated).
• Center MCP joints to IR, and adjust palmar surface of hand perpendicular to IR.
• Shield gonads.

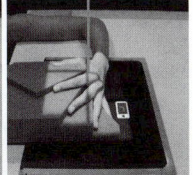

Central Ray
• Perpendicular to second MCP joint

Collimation:
1 inch (2.5 cm) on all sides of shadow of hand and thumb, including 1 inch (2.5 cm) proximal to ulnar styloid. Place side marker in the collimated exposure field.

kVp: 70   *Reference: 14th edition ATLAS p. 1:172.*

Manual Factors									
Part Thickness (cm)	mA	kVp	Time	mAs	SID	Image Receptor Size	CR, DR Exposure Indicator	Grid	HF, 1Ø or 3Ø

Notes: _____ Competency: ____/___/___

_____ Instructor: _____

Upper Extremity

Wrist
PA

Patient Position
• Seat patient at end of table with axilla in contact with table.

Part Position
• Have patient rest forearm on table.
• Center wrist to IR area.
• Flex digits slightly to place wrist in contact with IR.
• Shield gonads.

Central Ray
• Perpendicular to midcarpal area

Collimation:
2.5 inches (6 cm) proximal and distal to wrist joint and 1 inch (2.5 cm) on the sides. Place side marker in the collimated exposure field.

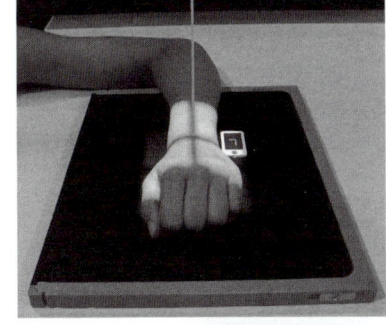

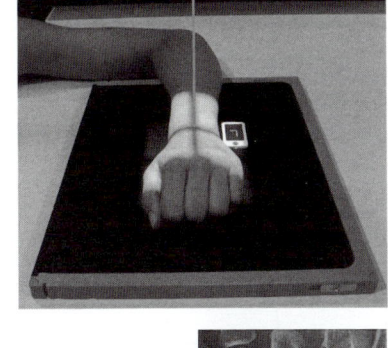

kVp: 66

Reference: 14th edition ATLAS p. 1:176.

Manual Factors									
Part Thickness (cm)	mA	kVp	Time	mAs	SID	Image Receptor Size	CR, DR Exposure Indicator	Grid	HF, 1Ø or 3Ø

Notes: _____ Competency: ____/____/____

_____ Instructor: _____

Upper Extremity

Wrist
Lateral

Patient Position
• Seat patient at end of table with axilla in contact with table.

Part Position
• Flex elbow 90 degrees, with forearm and arm in contact with table.
• Center carpals to IR, and adjust hand so that wrist is in true lateral position.
• Shield gonads.

Central Ray
• Perpendicular to wrist joint

Collimation:
2.5 inches (6 cm) proximal and distal to wrist joint and 1 inch (2.5 cm) on palmar and dorsal surfaces. Place side marker in the collimated exposure field.

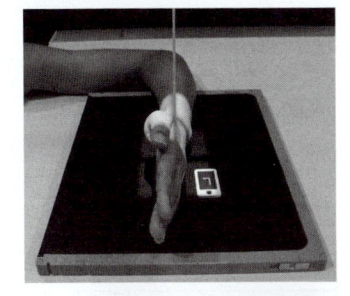

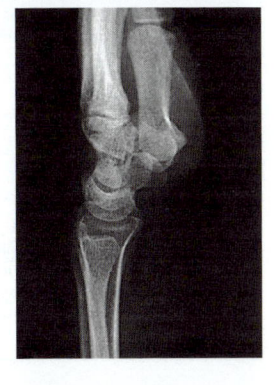

kVp: 70

Reference: 14th edition ATLAS p. 1:178.

Manual Factors									
Part Thickness (cm)	mA	kVp	Time	mAs	SID	Image Receptor Size	CR, DR Exposure Indicator	Grid	HF, 1Ø or 3Ø

Notes: _____ Competency: ____/____/____

_____ Instructor: _____

Upper Extremity

Wrist
PA oblique (lateral rotation)

Patient Position
• Seat patient at end of table with axilla in contact with table.

Part Position
• Rest anterior surface of wrist on IR.
• Center wrist to IR area.
• Rotate wrist approximately 45 degrees laterally (externally) and support on sponge.
• Shield gonads.

Central Ray
• Perpendicular to IR, entering midcarpal area just distal to radius

Collimation:
2.5 inches (6 cm) proximal and distal to wrist joint and 1 inch (2.5 cm) on sides. Place side marker in the collimated exposure field.

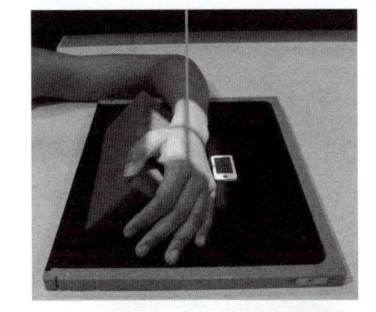

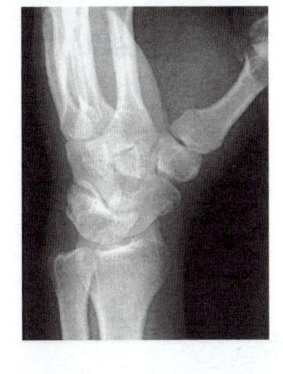

kVp: 66   *Reference: 14th edition ATLAS p. 1:180.*

Manual Factors									
Part Thickness (cm)	mA	kVp	Time	mAs	SID	Image Receptor Size	CR, DR Exposure Indicator	Grid	HF, 1Ø or 3Ø

Notes: _____ Competency: _____/___/___

_____ Instructor: _____

Upper Extremity

Wrist
PA: ulnar deviation

Patient Position
• Seat patient at end of table with axilla in contact with table.

Part Position
• Flex elbow 90 degrees, with forearm and arm in contact with table.
• Center wrist to IR area.
• Without moving the forearm, turn the hand outward until wrist is in extreme ulnar deviation.
• Shield gonads.

Central Ray
• Perpendicular to scaphoid

NOTE: If necessary to delineate fracture, angle central ray 10 to 15 degrees proximally (toward elbow) or distally.

Collimation:
2.5 inches (6 cm) proximal and distal to wrist joint and 1 inch (2.5 cm) on sides. Place side marker in the collimated exposure field.

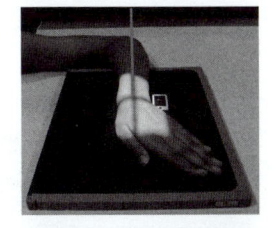

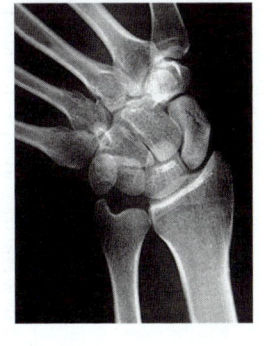

kVp: 66

Reference: 14th edition ATLAS p. 1:182.

Manual Factors									
Part Thickness (cm)	mA	kVp	Time	mAs	SID	Image Receptor Size	CR, DR Exposure Indicator	Grid	HF, 1Ø or 3Ø

Notes: _____ Competency: _____/___/___

_____ Instructor: _____

Upper Extremity

Wrist
PA axial STECHER METHOD

Patient Position
- Seat patient with arm and axilla in contact with table.

Part Position
- Place one end of IR on a support, and adjust so that finger end is elevated 20 degrees.
- Adjust the wrist for a PA projection, and center wrist to IR.
- Shield gonads.

Central Ray
- Perpendicular to table, and position to enter scaphoid

Collimation:
2½ inches (6 cm) proximal and distal to wrist joint and 1 inch (2.5 cm) on sides. Place side marker in the collimated exposure field.

kVp: 66

Reference: 14th edition ATLAS p. 1:184.

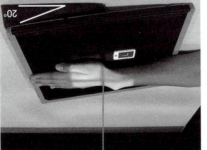
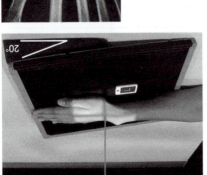

Manual Factors									
Part Thickness (cm)	mA	kVp	Time	mAs	SID	Image Receptor Size	CR, DR Exposure Indicator	Grid	HF, 1Ø or 3Ø

Notes: _____ Competency: _____/___/___

_____ Instructor: _____

Upper Extremity

Carpal Canal

Tangential GAYNOR-HART METHOD

Patient Position
- Seat patient with forearm parallel with long axis of table.

Part Position
- Hyperextend wrist, and center it to center of IR.
- Place ¾-inch radiolucent pad under lower forearm for support, if needed.
- Adjust hand position to make long axis of hand as vertical as possible.
- Have patient grasp digits with opposite hand to hold in extended position, or pull with a band (as shown).
- Shield gonads.

Central Ray
- Direct to palm of hand 1 inch (2.5 cm) distal to base of third metacarpal at 25- to 30-degree angle

Collimation:
1 inch (2.5 cm) on the three sides of shadow of wrist. Place side marker in the collimated exposure field.

kVp: 70 Reference: 14th edition ATLAS p. 1:190.

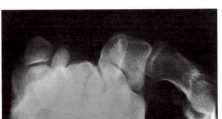

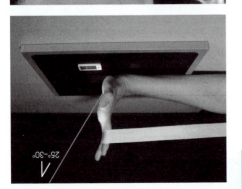

Manual Factors									
Part Thickness (cm)	mA	kVp	Time	mAs	SID	Image Receptor Size	CR, DR Exposure Indicator	Grid	HF, 1Ø or 3Ø

Notes: _____ Competency: ____/___/___

_____ Instructor: _____

Upper Extremity

Forearm
AP

Patient Position
- Seat patient at end of table with arm extended and entire extremity in same plane.

Part Position
- Supinate hand, and center forearm to IR to include joint or joints of interest.
- Adjust rotation to place humeral epicondyles equidistant from IR.
- Shield gonads.

Central Ray
- Perpendicular to midpoint of forearm

Collimation:
2 inches (5 cm) distal to wrist joint and proximal to elbow joint, and 1 inch (2.5 cm) on sides. Place side marker in the collimated exposure field.

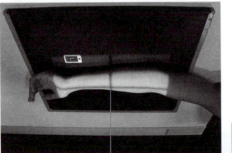
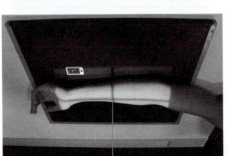

kVp: 70

Reference: 14th edition ATLAS p. 1:192.

Manual Factors										
Part Thickness (cm)	mA	kVp	Time	mAs	SID	Image Receptor Size	CR, DR Exposure Indicator	Grid	HF, 1Ø or 3Ø

Notes: _____ Competency: _____/___/___

_____ Instructor: _____

Upper Extremity

Forearm
Lateral

Patient Position
- Seat patient at end of table with humerus and forearm in contact with table.

Part Position
- Have patient flex elbow, and position entire extremity in same plane.
- Flex elbow 90 degrees, and adjust hand to lateral position (thumb up).
- Center forearm to IR to include joint or joints of interest.
- Shield gonads.

Central Ray
- Perpendicular to midpoint of forearm

Collimation:
2 inches (5 cm) distal to wrist joint and proximal to elbow joint, and 1 inch (2.5 cm) on sides. Place side marker in the collimated exposure field.

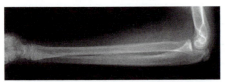

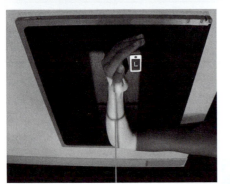

kVp: 70

Reference: 14th edition ATLAS p. 1:194.

Manual Factors									
Part Thickness (cm)	mA	kVp	Time	mAs	SID	Image Receptor Size	CR, DR Exposure Indicator	Grid	HF, 1Ø or 3Ø

Notes: _____ Competency: ____/____/____

_____ Instructor: _____

Upper Extremity

Elbow
AP

Patient Position
• Seat patient at end of table with arm extended and entire extremity in same plane.

Part Position
• Extend elbow, supinate hand, and center elbow joint to IR.
• Adjust humeral epicondyles to be equidistant from IR.
• Have patient lean slightly laterally if necessary to ensure AP alignment.
• Shield gonads.

Central Ray
• Perpendicular to elbow joint

Collimation:
3 inches (8 cm) proximal and distal to elbow joint and 1 inch (2.5 cm) on sides. Place side marker in the collimated exposure field.

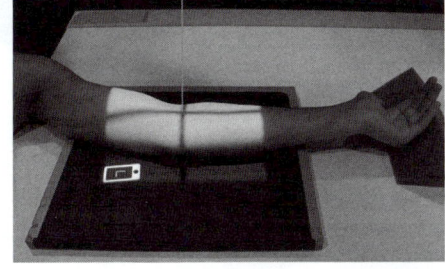

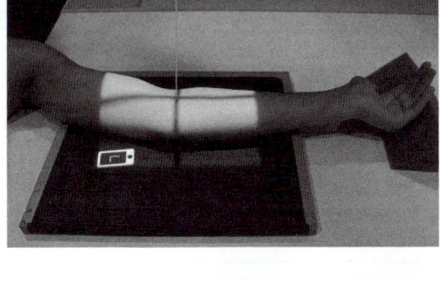

kVp: 70

Reference: 14th edition ATLAS p. 1:195.

Manual Factors									
Part Thickness (cm)	mA	kVp	Time	mAs	SID	Image Receptor Size	CR, DR Exposure Indicator	Grid	HF, 1Ø or 3Ø

Notes: _____ Competency: ____/____/____

_____ Instructor: _____

Upper Extremity

Elbow
Lateral

Patient Position
• Seat patient at end of table with elbow flexed 90 degrees.

Part Position
• Have patient rest humerus and forearm on table, and position entire extremity in same plane.
• Center 90-degree flexed elbow joint to IR, and adjust wrist and hand in lateral position.
• Adjust humeral epicondyles perpendicular to IR.
• Shield gonads.

Central Ray
• Perpendicular to elbow joint

Collimation:
3 inches (8 cm) proximal and distal to elbow joint. Place side marker in the collimated exposure field.

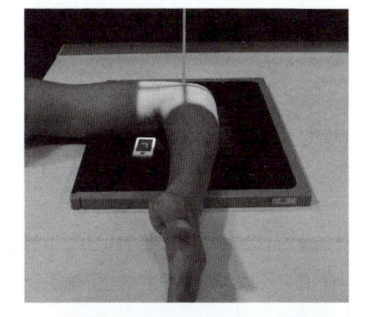

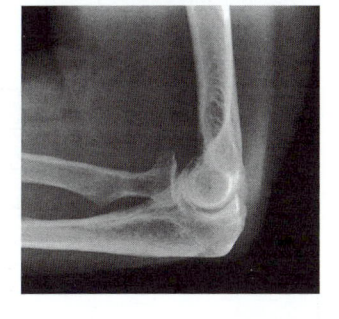

kVp: 70

Reference: 14th edition ATLAS p. 1:196.

Manual Factors									
Part Thickness (cm)	mA	kVp	Time	mAs	SID	Image Receptor Size	CR, DR Exposure Indicator	Grid	HF, 1Ø or 3Ø

Notes: _____ Competency: _____/___/___

_____ Instructor: _____

Upper Extremity

Elbow

AP oblique (medial rotation)

Patient Position
- Seat patient at end of table with arm extended and entire extremity in same plane.

Part Position
- Extend elbow, supinate hand, and center elbow joint to IR.
- Rotate arm medially.
- Adjust anterior surface of elbow (epicondyles) to 45 degrees to IR.
- Shield gonads.

Central Ray
- Perpendicular to IR, entering elbow joint

Collimation:
3 inches (8 cm) proximal and distal to elbow joint and 1 inch (2.5 cm) on sides. Place side marker in the collimated exposure field.

kVp: 70

Reference: 14th edition ATLAS p. 1:198.

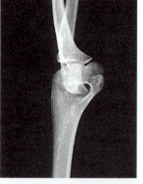

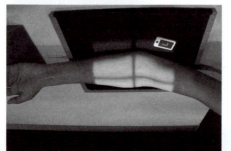

Manual Factors									
Part Thickness (cm)	mA	kVp	Time	mAs	SID	Image Receptor Size	CR, DR Exposure Indicator	Grid	HF, 1Ø or 3Ø

Notes: _____ Competency: _____/___/___

_____ Instructor: _____

Upper Extremity

Elbow
AP oblique (lateral rotation)

Patient Position
• Seat patient at end of table with arm extended and entire extremity in same plane.

Part Position
• Extend elbow, supinate hand, and center elbow joint to IR.
• Rotate arm laterally.
• Adjust anterior surface of elbow (epicondyles) to 45 degrees to IR.
• Shield gonads.

Central Ray
• Perpendicular to IR, entering elbow joint

Collimation:
3 inches (8 cm) proximal and distal to elbow joint and 1 inch (2.5 cm) on sides. Place side marker in the collimated exposure field.

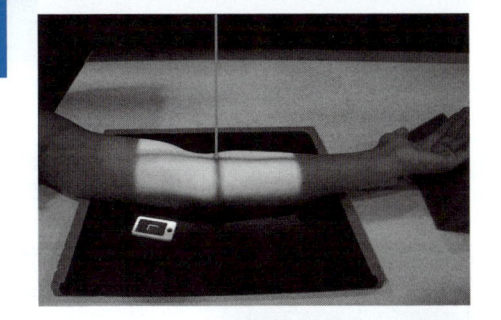

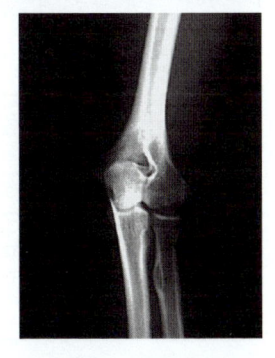

kVp: 70

Reference: 14th edition ATLAS p. 1:199.

Manual Factors									
Part Thickness (cm)	mA	kVp	Time	mAs	SID	Image Receptor Size	CR, DR Exposure Indicator	Grid	HF, 1Ø or 3Ø

Notes: _____ Competency: ____/____/____

_____ Instructor: _____

Upper Extremity

Elbow
AP partial flexion

Patient Position
- Seat patient at end of table with humerus resting on table for one image and forearm resting on table for the other image.

Part Position
Distal humerus:
- Place humerus on table, and support the elevated forearm.
- Support forearm.
- Supinate hand if possible.
- Place IR under elbow and center to condyloid area of the humerus.

Proximal forearm:
- Place dorsal surface of forearm on table.
- Place IR under elbow and center approximately 1 inch distal to humeral epicondyles.
- Shield gonads.

Central Ray
- Direct perpendicular to IR, entering appropriate portion of elbow joint

Collimation:
3 inches (8 cm) proximal and distal to elbow joint and 1 inch (2.5 cm) on sides. Place side marker in the collimated exposure field.

kVp: 70　　*Reference: 14th edition ATLAS pp 1-200-201*

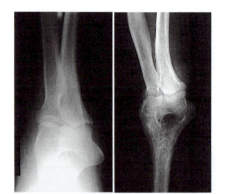
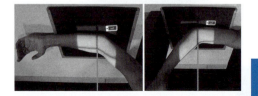

Manual Factors									
Part Thickness (cm)	mA	kVp	Time	mAs	SID	Image Receptor Size	CR, DR Exposure Indicator	Grid	HF, 1Ø or 3Ø

Notes: _____ Competency: ____/____/____

_____ Instructor: _____

Upper Extremity

Humerus
AP

Patient Position
• Position patient upright or supine.

Part Position
• Unless contraindicated, supinate hand.
• Adjust humerus with epicondyles parallel with IR.
• If patient is recumbent, elevate and support opposite shoulder, if needed.
• Center humerus to IR.
• Shield gonads.

Respiration:
• Obtain radiograph during suspended respiration.

Central Ray
• Perpendicular to midpoint of humerus

Collimation:
2 inches (5 cm) distal to elbow joint and superior to shoulder and 1 inch (2.5 cm) on sides. Place side marker in the collimated exposure field.

kVp: 70 (non-grid) 75 (grid)   *Reference: 14th edition ATLAS p. 1:211.*

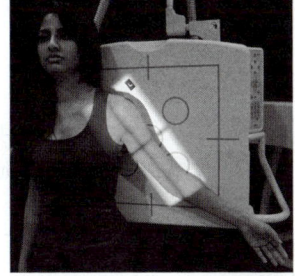
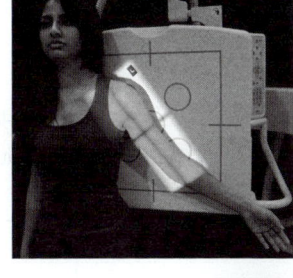

Manual Factors										
Part Thickness (cm)	mA	kVp	Time	mAs	SID	Image Receptor Size	CR, DR Exposure Indicator	Grid	HF, 1Ø or 3Ø

Notes: _____ Competency: ____/___/___

_____ Instructor: _____

Upper Extremity

Humerus
Lateral

Patient Position
• Position patient upright or supine.

Part Position
• Unless contraindicated, slightly abduct arm.
• Center arm to IR.
• Medially rotate arm until epicondyles are perpendicular to IR.
• Shield gonads.

Respiration:
• Suspend.

Central Ray
• Perpendicular to midpoint of humerus

Collimation:
2 inches (5 cm) distal to elbow joint and superior to shoulder and
1 inch (2.5 cm) on sides. Place side marker in the collimated exposure
field.

kVp: 70 (non-grid) 75 (grid)   *Reference: 14th edition ATLAS p. 1:214.*

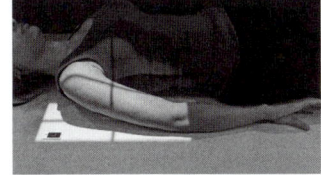
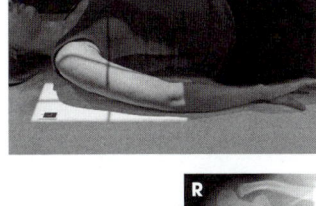

Manual Factors									
Part Thickness (cm)	mA	kVp	Time	mAs	SID	Image Receptor Size	CR, DR Exposure Indicator	Grid	HF, 1Ø or 3Ø

AEC Factors									
Part Thickness (cm)	mA	kVp	AEC Detector	mAs	Density Comp.	Image Receptor Size	CR, DR Exposure Indicator	Grid	HF, 1Ø or 3Ø

Notes: _____ Competency: ____/____/____

Instructor: _____

Upper Extremity

Proximal Humerus/Shoulder
Transthoracic lateral LAWRENCE METHOD

Patient Position
• Position patient upright or supine.

Part Position
• Raise uninjured arm, and rest it on or beside head.
• Elevate uninjured shoulder as much as possible.
• Adjust patient to project humerus between vertebral column and sternum.
• Unless contraindicated, adjust humeral epicondyles perpendicular to IR.

Respiration:
• Suspend.

Central Ray
• Perpendicular to midcoronal plane, exiting surgical neck of affected humerus. If patient cannot elevate unaffected shoulder, angle central ray 10 to 15 degrees cephalad.

Collimation:
Adjust to 10 × 12 inches (24 × 30 cm). Place side marker in the collimated exposure field.

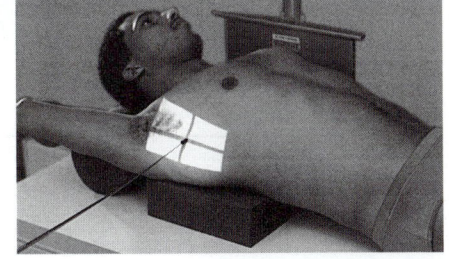

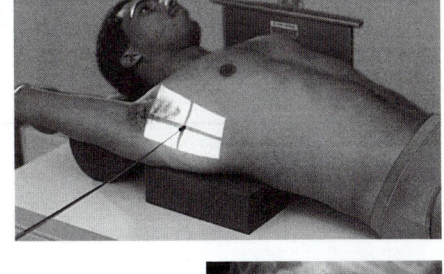

kVp: 85   *Reference: 14th edition ATLAS p. 1:236.*

Manual Factors									
Part Thickness (cm)	mA	kVp	Time	mAs	SID	Image Receptor Size	CR, DR Exposure Indicator	Grid	HF, 1Ø or 3Ø

AEC Factors									
Part Thickness (cm)	mA	kVp	AEC Detector	mAs	Density Comp.	Image Receptor Size	CR, DR Exposure Indicator	Grid	HF, 1Ø or 3Ø

Notes: _____ Competency: _____/_____/_____

_____ Instructor: _____

Upper Extremity

Shoulder
AP

Patient Position
- Position patient upright or supine.

Part Position
- Center a point 1 inch (2.5 cm) inferior to coracoid process to IR.
- Adjust hand in (1) external rotation: humeral epicondyles parallel to IR, (2) neutral rotation: epicondyles about 45 degrees to IR, or (3) internal rotation: epicondyles perpendicular to IR, depending on department protocol.
- Shield gonads.

Respiration:
- Suspend.

Central Ray
- Direct perpendicular to point 1 inch (2.5 cm) inferior to coracoid process

Collimation:
Adjust to 10 × 12 inches (24 × 30 cm). Place side marker in the collimated exposure field.

▼ COMPENSATING FILTER
- Shoulder filter greatly improves image quality.

kVp: 85   *Reference: 14th edition ATLAS p. 1:227*

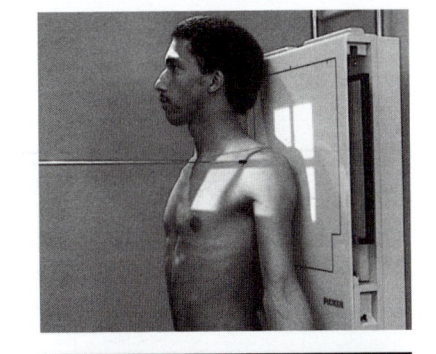

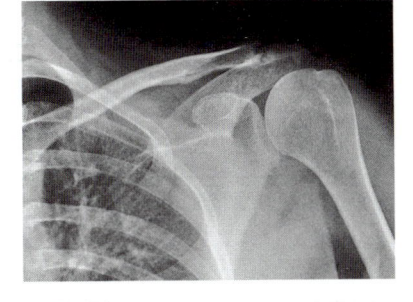

Manual Factors									
Part Thickness (cm)	mA	kVp	Time	mAs	SID	Image Receptor Size	CR, DR Exposure Indicator	Grid	HF, 1Ø or 3Ø

AEC Factors									
Part Thickness (cm)	mA	kVp	AEC Detector	mAs	Density Comp.	Image Receptor Size	CR, DR Exposure Indicator	Grid	HF, 1Ø or 3Ø

Notes: _____ Competency: ____/____/____

_____ Instructor: _____

Upper Extremity

Shoulder Joint
AP oblique   GRASHEY METHOD

Patient Position
• Position patient upright or recumbent.

Part Position
• Center IR to scapulohumeral joint. The joint is 2 inches (5 cm) medial and 2 inches (5 cm) inferior to superolateral border of shoulder.
• Rotate body 35 to 45 degrees toward affected side. (Note: Greater rotation may be needed to place plane of scapular body parallel to IR if patient is recumbent.)
• Abduct arm slightly with palm of hand on abdomen.
• Shield gonads.

Respiration:
• Suspend.

Central Ray
• Perpendicular to IR

Collimation:
Adjust to 8 × 10 inches (24 × 30 cm). Place side marker in the collimated exposure field.

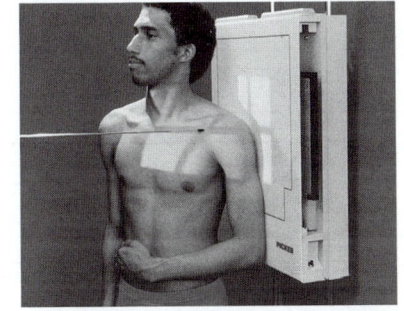
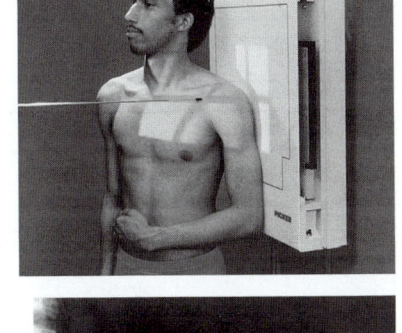

kVp: 85   *Reference: 14th edition ATLAS p. 1:232.*

Manual Factors									
Part Thickness (cm)	mA	kVp	Time	mAs	SID	Image Receptor Size	CR, DR Exposure Indicator	Grid	HF, 1Ø or 3Ø

AEC Factors									
Part Thickness (cm)	mA	kVp	AEC Detector	mAs	Density Comp.	Image Receptor Size	CR, DR Exposure Indicator	Grid	HF, 1Ø or 3Ø

Notes: _____ Competency: ___/___/___

Instructor: _____

Upper Extremity

Shoulder
Inferosuperior axial   LAWRENCE METHOD

Patient Position
- Position patient supine with head, affected shoulder, and elbow elevated 3 inches (8 cm).

Part Position
- Abduct affected arm 90 degrees from body, if possible.
- Keep arm in external rotation, and support on pillow or sandbags.
- Place vertically oriented IR above shoulder as close to neck as possible.
- Turn patient's head away from side being examined.
- Shield gonads.

Respiration:
- Suspend.

Central Ray
- Horizontally through axilla to exit region of acromioclavicular joint. Direct 15 to 30 degrees medially.

Collimation:
Adjust 12 inches (30 cm) in length and 1 inch (2.5 cm) above anterior shadow of shoulder. Place side marker in the collimated exposure field.

kVp: 75

Reference: 14th edition ATLAS p. 1:238.

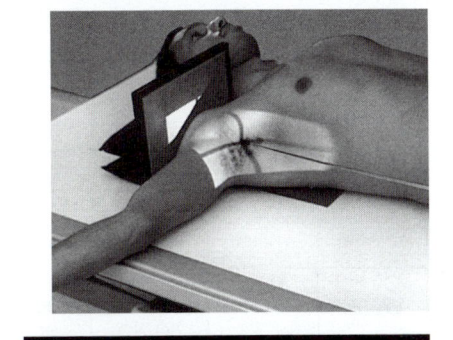

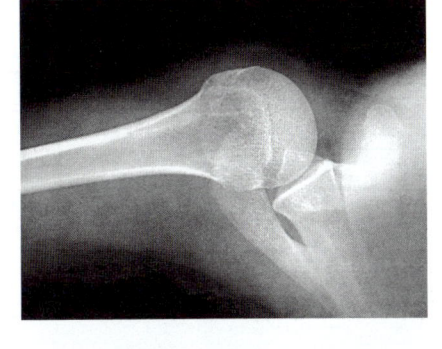

Manual Factors

Part Thickness (cm)	mA	kVp	Time	mAs	SID	Image Receptor Size	CR, DR Exposure Indicator	Grid	HF, 1Ø or 3Ø

AEC Factors

Part Thickness (cm)	mA	kVp	AEC Detector	mAs	Density Comp.	Image Receptor Size	CR, DR Exposure Indicator	Grid	HF, 1Ø or 3Ø

Notes: _____

Competency: ____/____/____

Instructor: _____

Upper Extremity

Shoulder (Scapular Y)
PA oblique

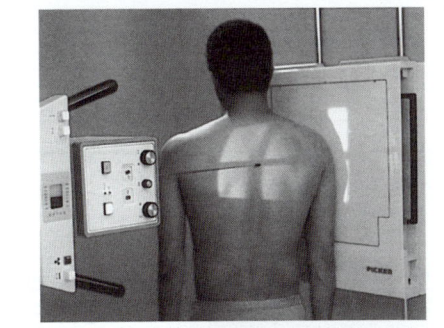

Patient Position
• Position patient upright or prone. Upright position is preferred when shoulder is tender.

Part Position
• Center anterior surface of affected shoulder to IR.
• Palpate scapular borders, and rotate patient so that midcoronal plane forms 45- to 60-degree angle from IR. (Note: Plane of scapular body will be perpendicular to IR.)
• Shield gonads.

Respiration:
• Suspend.

Central Ray
• Perpendicular to shoulder joint at level of scapulohumeral joint

Collimation:
Adjust to 12 inches (30 cm) in length and 1 inch (2.5 cm) to lateral shadow. Place side marker in the collimated exposure field.

◥ COMPENSATING FILTER
• Shoulder filter greatly improves radiographic quality.

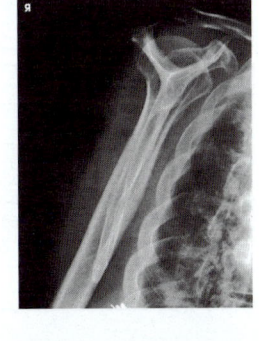

kVp: 85   *Reference: 14th edition ATLAS p. 1:243.*

Manual Factors

Part Thickness (cm)	mA	kVp	Time	mAs	SID	Image Receptor Size	CR, DR Exposure Indicator	Grid	HF, 1Ø or 3Ø

AEC Factors

Part Thickness (cm)	mA	kVp	AEC Detector	mAs	Density Comp.	Image Receptor Size	CR, DR Exposure Indicator	Grid	HF, 1Ø or 3Ø

Notes: _____ Competency: _____/___/___

Instructor: _____

Upper Extremity

Acromioclavicular Articulations
AP PEARSON METHOD

Patient Position
• Position patient upright if condition permits.

Part Position
• Adjust midpoint of IR to level of acromioclavicular (AC) joints.
• Center midsagittal plane of body to midline of IR if both AC joints can be shown on one radiograph. Otherwise, center to each individual AC joint for two separate exposures.
• To show AC separation, attach sandbags of equal weight (5–10 lb) to each wrist and also obtain a second radiograph without weights for comparison.

Respiration:
• Suspend.

Central Ray
• Perpendicular to IR midway between AC joints (for one exposure) or perpendicular to each AC joint (for two exposures)

Collimation:
Adjust to 6 × 17 inches (15 × 43 cm) for single exposure or 3.5 × 3.5 inches (9 × 9 cm) for two exposures. Place side marker in the collimated exposure field.

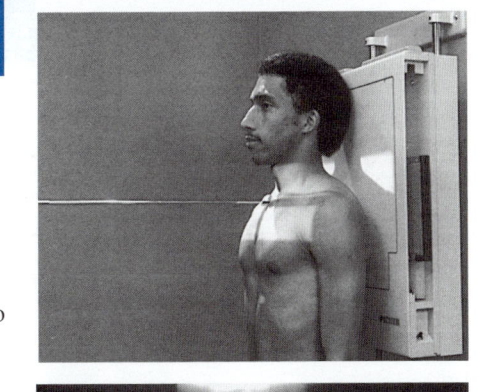

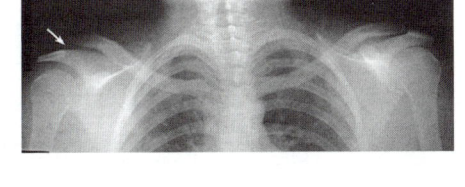

kVp: 80   Reference: 14th edition ATLAS p. 1:253

Manual Factors

Part Thickness (cm)	mA	kVp	Time	mAs	SID	Image Receptor Size	CR, DR Exposure Indicator	Grid	HF, 1Ø or 3Ø

AEC Factors

Part Thickness (cm)	mA	kVp	AEC Detector	mAs	Density Comp.	Image Receptor Size	CR, DR Exposure Indicator	Grid	HF, 1Ø or 3Ø

Notes: _____ Competency: ____/____/____

_____ Instructor: _____

Upper Extremity

Clavicle
AP

Patient Position
• Position patient upright or supine.

Part Position
• Center clavicle to center of IR, midway between midline of body and lateral border of shoulder.
• Turn patient's head away from affected side.
• Shield gonads.

Respiration:
• Suspend.

Central Ray
• Perpendicular to midshaft of clavicle
NOTE: If necessary to decrease part-IR distance and to improve recorded detail, obtain PA clavicle. Place patient facing grid using perpendicular central ray, and position using above-mentioned landmarks.

Collimation:
Adjust to 8 × 12 inches (18 × 30 cm). Place side marker in the collimated exposure field.

kVp: 80

Reference: 14th edition ATLAS p. 1:257.

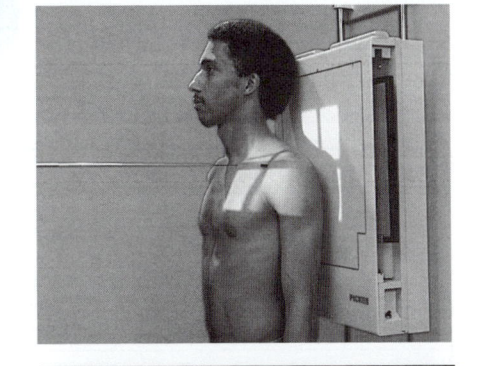

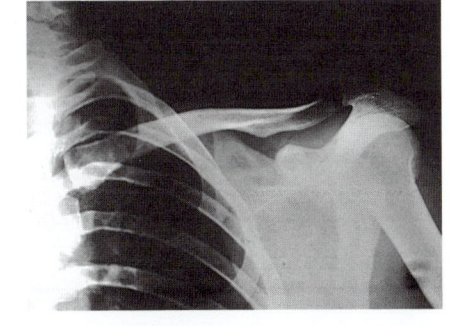

Manual Factors									
Part Thickness (cm)	mA	kVp	Time	mAs	SID	Image Receptor Size	CR, DR Exposure Indicator	Grid	HF, 1Ø or 3Ø

AEC Factors									
Part Thickness (cm)	mA	kVp	AEC Detector	mAs	Density Comp.	Image Receptor Size	CR, DR Exposure Indicator	Grid	HF, 1Ø or 3Ø

Notes: _____ Competency: _____/_____/_____

Instructor: _____

Upper Extremity

Clavicle
AP axial

Patient Position
• Position patient upright or supine.

Part Position
• Center clavicle to lower third of IR, midway between midsagittal plane and lateral border of shoulder.
• Turn patient's head away from affected side if necessary.
• Shield gonads.

Respiration:
• Suspend.

Central Ray
• Angled 15 to 30 degrees cephalad centered to midshaft of clavicle
NOTE: If necessary to decrease part-IR distance and to improve recorded detail, obtain PA axial clavicle. Place patient facing grid using 15 to 20 degrees caudal central ray angulation.

Collimation:
Adjust to 8 × 12 inches (18 × 30 cm). Place side marker in the collimated exposure field.

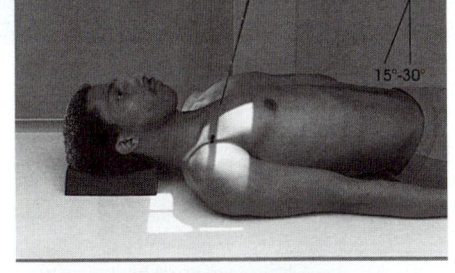

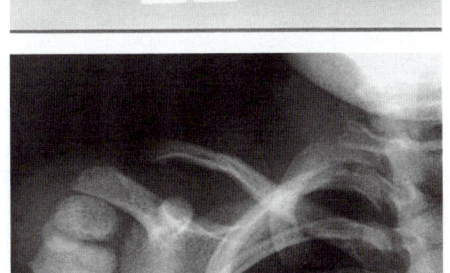

kVp: 80

Reference: 14th edition ATLAS p. 1:258.

Manual Factors									
Part Thickness (cm)	mA	kVp	Time	mAs	SID	Image Receptor Size	CR, DR Exposure Indicator	Grid	HF, 1Ø or 3Ø

AEC Factors									
Part Thickness (cm)	mA	kVp	AEC Detector	mAs	Density Comp.	Image Receptor Size	CR, DR Exposure Indicator	Grid	HF, 1Ø or 3Ø

Notes: _____ Competency: ____/____/____

_____ Instructor: _____

Upper Extremity

Scapula
AP

Patient Position
• Position patient supine or upright. Upright position is preferred when shoulder is tender.

Part Position
• Abduct arm to a right angle to body, flex elbow, and support hand.
• Center palpated scapular area to IR approximately 2 inches (5 cm) inferior to coracoid process.
• Shield gonads.

Respiration:
• Slow breathing.

Central Ray
• Perpendicular to IR at mid-scapular area approximately 2 inches (5 cm) inferior to coracoid process

Collimation:
Adjust to 10 × 12 inches (24 × 30 cm). Place side marker in the collimated exposure field.

kVp: 85

Reference: 14th edition ATLAS p. 1:260.

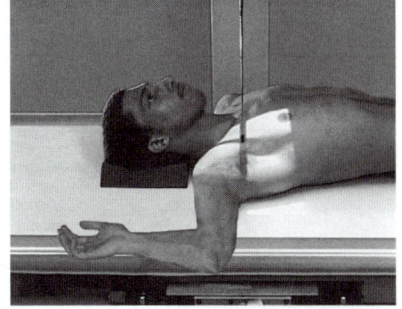
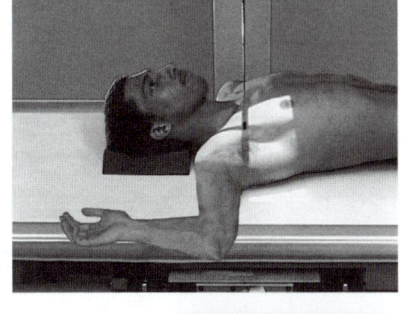

Manual Factors

Part Thickness (cm)	mA	kVp	Time	mAs	SID	Image Receptor Size	CR, DR Exposure Indicator	Grid	HF, 1Ø or 3Ø

AEC Factors

Part Thickness (cm)	mA	kVp	AEC Detector	mAs	Density Comp.	Image Receptor Size	CR, DR Exposure Indicator	Grid	HF, 1Ø or 3Ø

Notes: _____ Competency: ____/____/____

Instructor: _____

Upper Extremity

Scapula
Lateral

Patient Position
- Position patient prone or upright. Upright position is preferred when shoulder is tender.

Part Position
- Place patient in oblique position 45 to 60 degrees, and center affected scapula to IR.
- Extend affected arm across anterior or posterior thorax or above head to show appropriate portion of scapula.
- Palpate medial and lateral borders of scapula, and adjust body rotation so that scapula is lateral and is projected free of rib cage.
- Shield gonads.

Respiration:
- Suspend.

Central Ray
- Perpendicular to IR, and position to medial border of protruding scapula

Collimation:
Adjust to 12 inches (30 cm) in length and 1 inch (2.5 cm) to lateral shadow. Place side marker in the collimated exposure field.

▼ COMPENSATING FILTER
- Shoulder filter greatly improves radiographic quality.

kVp: 85 *Reference: 14th edition ATLAS p. 1:262*

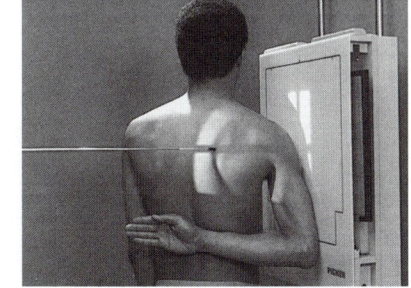

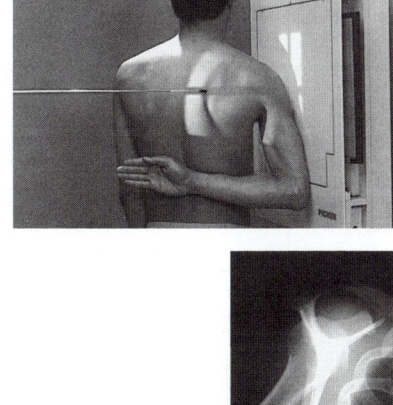

Manual Factors

Part Thickness (cm)	mA	kVp	Time	mAs	SID	Image Receptor Size	CR, DR Exposure Indicator	Grid	HF, 1Ø or 3Ø

AEC Factors

Part Thickness (cm)	mA	kVp	AEC Detector	mAs	Density Comp.	Image Receptor Size	CR, DR Exposure Indicator	Grid	HF, 1Ø or 3Ø

Notes: _____

Competency: _____/____/____

Instructor: _____

Upper Extremity

Toes:
  AP or AP axial, 72
  AP oblique (medial rotation), 74
  Lateral, 76
Foot:
  AP or AP axial, 78
  AP oblique (medial rotation), 80
  Lateral (mediolateral), 82
Calcaneus:
  Axial (plantar dorsal), 84
  Lateral, 86
Ankle:
  AP, 88
  Lateral (mediolateral), 90
  AP oblique (medial rotation), 92
Ankle (Mortise Joint):
  AP oblique (medial rotation), 94
  AP stress studies, 96

Leg:
  AP, 98
  Lateral, 100
Knee:
  AP, 102
  AP weight-bearing, 104
  Lateral, 106
  AP oblique (lateral rotation), 108
  AP oblique (medial rotation), 110
Intercondylar Fossa:
  PA axial; HOLMBLAD METHOD, 112
  PA axial; CAMP-COVENTRY METHOD, 114
Patella:
  PA, 116
  Lateral (mediolateral), 118
  Tangential; SETTEGAST METHOD, 120

Femur:
  AP, 122
  Lateral, 124
Femoral Necks:
  AP oblique; MODIFIED CLEAVES METHOD, 126
Hip:
  AP, 128
  Lateral; LAUENSTEIN AND HICKEY METHODS, 130
  Axiolateral; DANELIUS-MILLER METHOD, 132
Pelvis and Upper Femora:
  AP, 134

Lower Extremity

Toes
AP or AP axial

Patient Position
- Position patient supine or seated on table, knees flexed with feet separated.

Part Position
- Center toes with plantar surface flat against IR.
- Shield gonads.

Central Ray
- Angle 15 degrees posteriorly to show joint spaces.
- Position so that central ray enters third MTP joint.
- Use perpendicular central ray when joint spaces are not crucial.

Collimation:
1 inch (2.5 cm) on all sides of toes including 1 inch (2.5 cm) proximal to MTP joint. Place side marker in the collimated exposure field.

▼ COMPENSATING FILTER
- Image can be improved significantly with use of filter.

kVp: 63

Reference: 14th edition ATLAS p. 1:288.

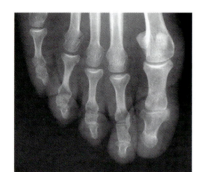
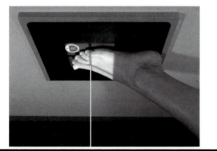

Manual Factors

Part Thickness (cm)	mA	kVp	Time	mAs	SID	Image Receptor Size	CR, DR Exposure Indicator	Grid	HF, 1Ø or 3Ø

Notes: _____ Competency: _____/___/___

_____ Instructor: _____

Lower Extremity

Toes
AP oblique (medial rotation)

Patient Position
• Position patient supine or seated on table, knees flexed with feet separated.

Part Position
• Center toes over IR area, and medially rotate leg and foot until 30- to 45-degree angle is formed from IR to plantar surface of foot.
• Shield gonads.

Central Ray
• Perpendicular, entering third MTP joint

Collimation:
1 inch (2.5 cm) on all sides of toes including 1 inch (2.5 cm) proximal to MTP joint. Place side marker in the collimated exposure field.

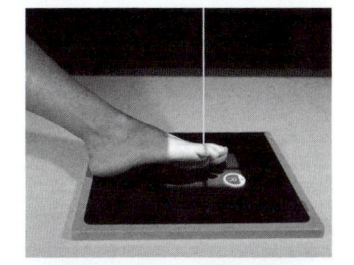

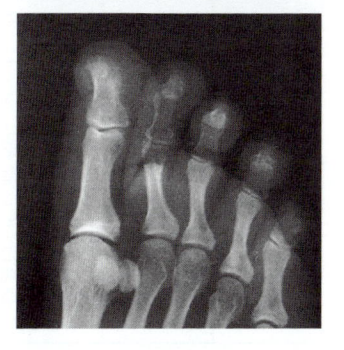

kVp: 63

Reference: 14th edition ATLAS p. 1:291.

Manual Factors									
Part Thickness (cm)	mA	kVp	Time	mAs	SID	Image Receptor Size	CR, DR Exposure Indicator	Grid	HF, 1Ø or 3Ø

Notes: _____

Competency: _____/___/___

Instructor: _____

Lower Extremity

Toes
Lateral

Patient Position
- Position patient on unaffected side (for great and second toes) or affected side (for third through fifth toes).

Part Position
- Adjust foot to place affected toe parallel to IR and in true lateral position.
- Use gauze, tape, or other positioning aid to separate toes.
- Shield gonads.

Central Ray
- Perpendicular to IP joint of great toe or PIP joint of second through fifth toes

Collimation:
1 inch (2.5 cm) on all sides of toe including 1 inch (2.5 cm) proximal to joint. Place side marker in the collimated exposure field.

kVp: 63

Reference: 14th edition ATLAS p. 1:292.

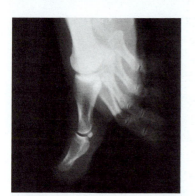
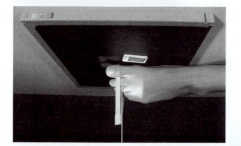

Manual Factors									
Part Thickness (cm)	mA	kVp	Time	mAs	SID	Image Receptor Size	CR, DR Exposure Indicator	Grid	HF, 1Ø or 3Ø

Notes: _____

Competency: _____/___/___

Instructor: _____

Lower Extremity

Foot
AP or AP axial

Patient Position
- Position patient supine or seated on table, knees flexed with feet separated.

Part Position
- Place plantar surface of foot in center of IR, and adjust midline of foot parallel to long axis of IR.
- Shield gonads.

Central Ray
- Angle 10 degrees toward the heel (posteriorly), entering base of third metatarsal.
- Direct perpendicularly, if dictated by department protocol.

Collimation:
1 inch (2.5 cm) on sides and 1 inch (2.5 cm) beyond the calcaneus and distal tip of toes. Place side marker in the collimated exposure field.

COMPENSATING FILTER
- Image can be improved significantly with use of filter.

kVp: 70

Reference: 14th edition ATLAS p. 1:298.

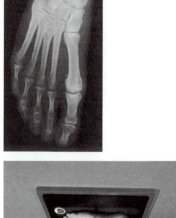
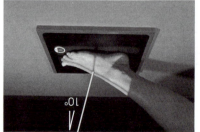

Manual Factors

Part Thickness (cm)	mA	kVp	Time	mAs	SID	Image Receptor Size	CR, DR Exposure Indicator	Grid	HF, 1Ø or 3Ø

Notes: _____ Competency: _____/_____/_____

_____ Instructor: _____

Lower Extremity

Foot
AP oblique (medial rotation)

Patient Position
• Position patient supine or seated on table, knees flexed with feet separated.

Part Position
• Center foot to IR.
• Rotate leg medially until plantar surface of foot forms angle of 30 degrees to IR.
• Shield gonads.

Central Ray
• Perpendicular to base of third metatarsal

Collimation:
1 inch (2.5 cm) on sides and 1 inch (2.5 cm) beyond the calcaneus and distal tip of toes. Place side marker in the collimated exposure field.

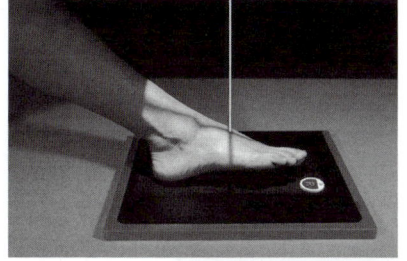

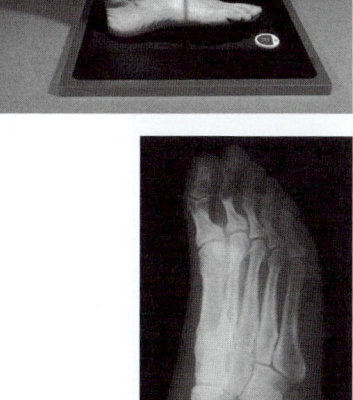

kVp: 70   *Reference: 14th edition ATLAS p. 1:302.*

Manual Factors										
Part Thickness (cm)	mA	kVp	Time	mAs	SID	Image Receptor Size	CR, DR Exposure Indicator	Grid	HF, 1Ø or 3Ø

Notes: _____

Competency: _____/____/____

Instructor: _____

Lower Extremity

Foot
Lateral (mediolateral)

Patient Position
- Position patient on affected side.

Part Position
- Center foot to IR and adjust plantar surface perpendicular to IR.
- Adjust leg and foot in lateral position with patella perpendicular to table.
- Dorsiflex foot to form 90-degree angle with lower leg.
- Shield gonads.

Central Ray
- Perpendicular to midpoint of IR, entering level of base of third metatarsal

Collimation:
1 inch (2.5 cm) on all sides of shadow of foot, including 1 inch (2.5 cm) above medial malleolus. Place side marker in the collimated exposure field.

kVp: 70

Reference: 14th edition ATLAS p. 1:306.

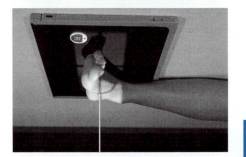
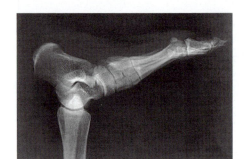

Manual Factors

Part Thickness (cm)	mA	kVp	Time	mAs	SID	Image Receptor Size	CR, DR Exposure Indicator	Grid	HF, 1Ø or 3Ø

Notes: _____ Competency: _____/___/___

_____ Instructor: _____

Lower Extremity

Calcaneus
Axial (plantodorsal)

Patient Position
- Position patient supine or seated with leg fully extended.

Part Position
- Center IR to ankle.
- Have patient dorsiflex foot to place plantar surface perpendicular to IR.
- Shield gonads.

Central Ray
- Angle 40 degrees cephalad to long axis of foot so that central ray enters plantar surface of foot at base of third metatarsal.

Collimation:
1 inch (2.5 cm) on three sides of shadow of calcaneus. Place side marker in the collimated exposure field.

COMPENSATING FILTER
- Image can be improved significantly with use of filter.

kVp: 70

Reference: 14th edition ATLAS p. 1:317.

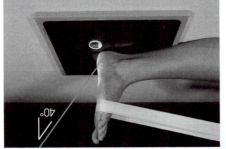
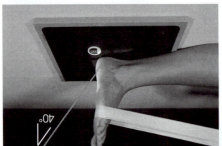

Manual Factors									
Part Thickness (cm)	mA	kVp	Time	mAs	SID	Image Receptor Size	CR, DR Exposure Indicator	Grid	HF, 1Ø or 3Ø

Notes: _____

Competency: _____/_____/_____

Instructor: _____

Lower Extremity

Calcaneus
Lateral

Patient Position
- Position patient on affected side.

Part Position
- Center calcaneus to center of IR.
- Adjust leg and foot in lateral position with patella perpendicular to table.

Central Ray
- Perpendicular to midportion of calcaneus, about 1 inch (2.5 cm) distal to medial malleolus.

Collimation:
1 inch (2.5 cm) past posterior and inferior shadow of heel; include medial malleolus and base of fifth metatarsal. Place side marker in the collimated exposure field.

kVp: 70

Reference: 14th edition ATLAS p. 1:320.

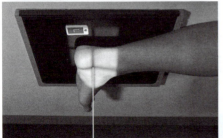

Manual Factors

Part Thickness (cm)	mA	kVp	Time	mAs	SID	Image Receptor Size	CR, DR Exposure Indicator	Grid	HF, 1Ø or 3Ø

Notes: _____ Competency: _____/___/___

_____ Instructor: _____

Lower Extremity

Ankle
AP

kVp: 70   *Reference: 14th edition ATLAS p. 1:325.*

Patient Position
- Position patient supine or seated on table with affected leg extended.

Part Position
- Center ankle to IR.
- Adjust ankle joint in anatomic position to obtain true AP projection.
- Have patient flex foot, and adjust ankle with toes pointing vertically.

Central Ray
- Perpendicular to ankle joint, entering midway between malleoli.

Collimation:
- 1 inch (2.5 cm) on sides of ankle and 8 inches (18 cm) lengthwise, including heel. Place side marker in the collimated exposure field.

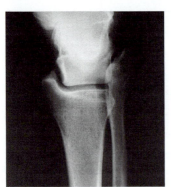
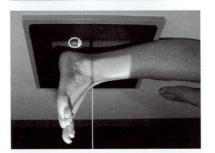

Manual Factors

Part Thickness (cm)	mA	kVp	Time	mAs	SID	Image Receptor Size	CR, DR Exposure Indicator	Grid	HF, 1Ø or 3Ø

Notes: _____ Competency: _____/____/____

_____ Instructor: _____

Lower Extremity

kVp: 70 Reference: 14th edition ATLAS p. 1:326.

Ankle
Lateral (mediolateral)

Patient Position
- Position patient supine, then roll onto affected side.

Part Position
- Center ankle to IR.
- Dorsiflex ankle to 90-degree angle, and adjust foot in lateral position.

Central Ray
- Perpendicular to ankle joint, entering medial malleolus.

Collimation:
1 inch (2.5 cm) on sides of ankle and 8 inches (18 cm) lengthwise, including heel and fifth metacarpal base. Place side marker in the collimated exposure field.

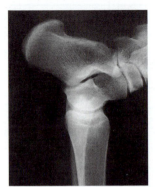
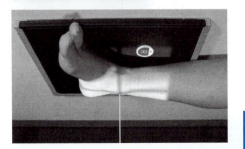

Manual Factors

Part Thickness (cm)	mA	kVp	Time	mAs	SID	Image Receptor Size	CR, DR Exposure Indicator	Grid	HF, 1Ø or 3Ø

Notes: _____

Competency: _____/___/___

Instructor: _____

Lower Extremity

Ankle
AP oblique (medial rotation)

Patient Position
- Position patient supine or seated on table.

Part Position
- Center ankle to IR.
- Dorsiflex foot, placing ankle at near right-angle flexion.
- Internally rotate entire leg and foot together until 45-degree rotation is achieved.

Central Ray
- Perpendicular to ankle joint, entering midway between malleoli.

Collimation:
- 1 inch (2.5 cm) on sides of ankle and 8 inches (18 cm) lengthwise, including heel. Place side marker in the collimated exposure field.

NOTE: Obtain lateral rotation oblique by rotating leg and foot 45 degrees laterally, as described in 14th edition ATLAS p. 1:xxx.

kVp: 70

Reference: 14th edition ATLAS p. 1:329.

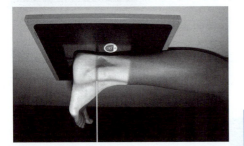
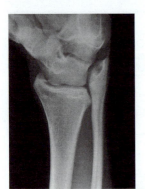

Manual Factors

Part Thickness (cm)	mA	kVp	Time	mAs	SID	Image Receptor Size	CR, DR Exposure Indicator	Grid	HF, 1Ø or 3Ø

Notes: _____ Competency: _____/___/___

_____ Instructor: _____

Lower Extremity

Ankle (Mortise Joint)
AP oblique (medial rotation)

Patient Position
• Position patient supine or seated on table.

Part Position
• Center ankle to IR.
• Dorsiflex foot, placing ankle at near right-angle flexion.
• Medially rotate entire leg and foot together 15 to 20 degrees until intermalleolar plane is parallel to IR.

Central Ray
• Perpendicular, entering ankle joint midway between malleoli.

Collimation:
1 inch (2.5 cm) on sides of ankle and 8 inches (18 cm) lengthwise, including heel. Place side marker in the collimated exposure field.

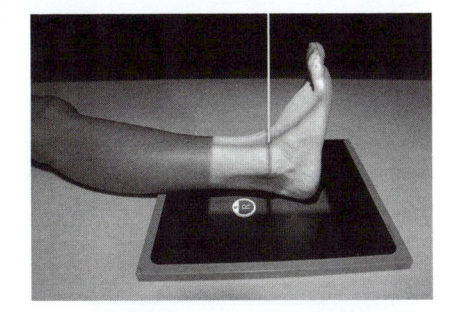

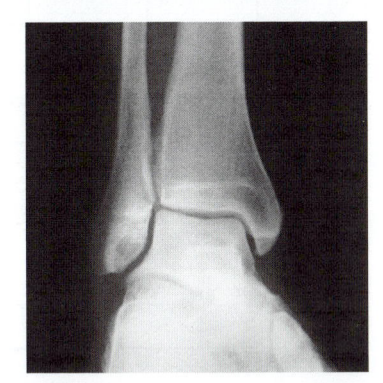

kVp: 70

Reference: 14th edition ATLAS p. 1:330.

Manual Factors									
Part Thickness (cm)	mA	kVp	Time	mAs	SID	Image Receptor Size	CR, DR Exposure Indicator	Grid	HF, 1Ø or 3Ø

Notes: _____   Competency: _____/____/____

_____   Instructor: _____

Lower Extremity

Ankle
AP stress studies

Patient Position
• Position patient supine or seated on table with small support under knee.

Part Position
• Center ankle to IR.
• Position ankle for AP projection.
• Stress joint by placing it in position of extreme inversion or eversion, then immobilizing it.

Central Ray
• Perpendicular to ankle joint, entering midway between malleoli.

Collimation:
1 inch (2.5 cm) on sides of ankle and 8 inches (18 cm) lengthwise, including heel. Place side marker in the collimated exposure field.

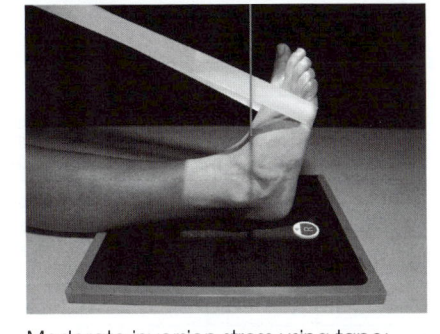

Moderate inversion stress using tape; lead glove recommended for increased stress.

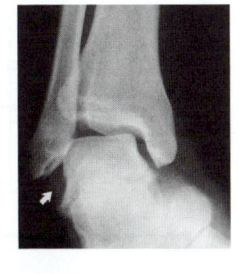

kVp: 70   *Reference: 14th edition ATLAS p. 1:333.*

Manual Factors

Part Thickness (cm)	mA	kVp	Time	mAs	SID	Image Receptor Size	CR, DR Exposure Indicator	Grid	HF, 1Ø or 3Ø

Notes: _____ Competency: _____/___/___

_____ Instructor: _____

Lower Extremity

Leg
AP

Patient Position
- Position patient supine with leg extended.

Part Position
- Center leg to IR, and adjust leg so that femoral condyles are parallel to IR and foot is vertical; flex ankle to 90 degrees.
- Include both joints.

Central Ray
- Perpendicular to midpoint of leg.

Collimation:
1 inch (2.5 cm) on sides and 1.5 inches (3.8 cm) beyond the ankle and knee joints. Place side marker in the collimated exposure field.

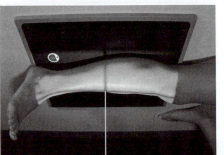

kVp: 70 (non-grid), 80 (grid)   *Reference: 14th edition ATLAS p. 1:336.*

Manual Factors										
Part Thickness (cm)	mA	kVp	Time	mAs	SID	Image Receptor Size	CR, DR Exposure Indicator	Grid	HF, 1Ø or 3Ø

Notes: _____ Competency: ____/____/____

Instructor: _____

Lower Extremity

Leg
Lateral

Patient Position
- Position patient supine on affected side.

Part Position
- Center leg to IR.
- Adjust leg to lateral position (patella perpendicular).
- Include both joints.

Central Ray
- Perpendicular to midpoint of leg.

Collimation:
1 inch (2.5 cm) on sides and 1.5 inches (3.8 cm) beyond the ankle and knee joints. Place side marker in the collimated exposure field.

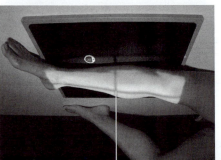
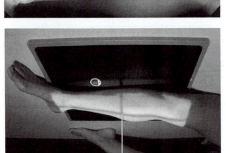

kVp: 70 (non-grid), 80 (grid)   *Reference: 14th edition ATLAS p. 1:338.*

Manual Factors									
Part Thickness (cm)	mA	kVp	Time	mAs	SID	Image Receptor Size	CR, DR Exposure Indicator	Grid	HF, 1Ø or 3Ø

Notes: _____ Competency: _____/_____/_____

_____ Instructor: _____

Lower Extremity

Knee
AP

Patient Position
- Position patient supine with leg extended.
- Adjust patient's body so that pelvis is not rotated.

Part Position
- Center knee to IR at level ½ inch (1.3 cm) below patellar apex.
- Adjust leg so that femoral condyles are parallel to IR.

Central Ray
- Enters point ½ inch (1.3 cm) inferior to patellar apex.
- Depending on ASIS-to-tabletop measurement, direct central ray as follows:

<19 cm	3 to 5 degrees *caudad* (thin pelvis)
19 to 24 cm	0 degrees
>24 cm	3 to 5 degrees *cephalad* (large pelvis)

Collimation:
Adjust to 8 × 10 inches (18 × 24 cm). Adjust to 1 inch (2.5 cm) beyond the sides. Place side marker in the collimated exposure field.

kVp: 70 (non-grid), 85 (grid)   Reference: 14th edition ATLAS p. 1:342.

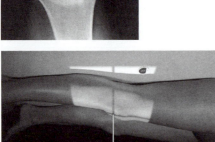

Manual Factors

Part Thickness (cm)	mA	kVp	Time	mAs	SID	Image Receptor Size	CR, DR Exposure Indicator	Grid	HF, 1Ø or 3Ø

AEC Factors

Part Thickness (cm)	mA	kVp	AEC Detector	mAs	Density Comp.	Image Receptor Size	CR, DR Exposure Indicator	Grid	HF, 1Ø or 3Ø

Notes: _____ Competency: ____/____/____

_____ Instructor: _____

Lower Extremity

Knee
AP weight-bearing

Patient Position
• Position patient upright facing x-ray tube with weight equally distributed on feet.

Part Position
• Adjust center of IR ½ inch (1.3 cm) below level of patellar apices.
• Have patient point toes straight ahead and slightly separate knees.

Central Ray
• Horizontal and perpendicular to IR, entering midway between knees at level ½ inch (1.3 cm) below patellar apices.

Collimation:
Adjust to 14 × 17 inches (35 × 43 cm). Place side marker in the collimated exposure field.

kVp: 70 (non-grid), 85 (grid)   *Reference: 14th edition ATLAS p. 1:348.*

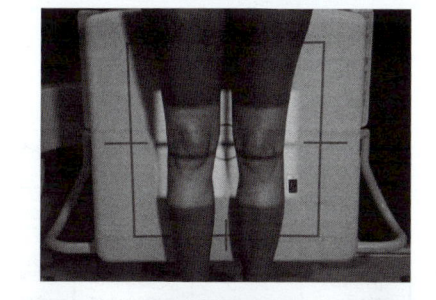

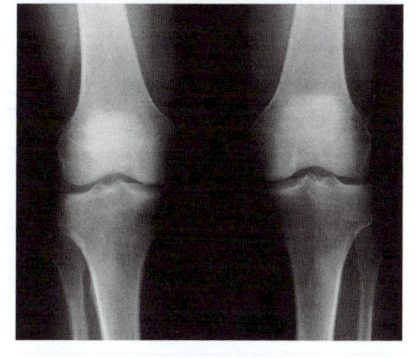

Manual Factors									
Part Thickness (cm)	mA	kVp	Time	mAs	SID	Image Receptor Size	CR, DR Exposure Indicator	Grid	HF, 1Ø or 3Ø

AEC Factors									
Part Thickness (cm)	mA	kVp	AEC Detector	mAs	Density Comp.	Image Receptor Size	CR, DR Exposure Indicator	Grid	HF, 1Ø or 3Ø

Notes: _____ Competency: ____/____/____

Instructor: _____

Lower Extremity

Knee
Lateral

Patient Position
- Position patient recumbent on affected side.

Part Position
- Have patient flex knee 20 to 30 degrees, and center IR to knee joint, just below patellar apex.
- Position patella perpendicular to IR.

Central Ray
- Angle 5 to 7 degrees cephalad, entering knee joint 1 inch (2.5 cm) distal to medial epicondyle.

Collimation:
Adjust to 8 × 10 inch (18 × 24 cm). Adjust to 1 inch (2.5 cm) anterior to the patella and 1 inch (2.5 cm) beyond the posterior shadow. Place side marker in the collimated exposure field.

kVp: 70 (non-grid), 85 (grid)   *Reference: 14th edition ATLAS p. 1:346.*

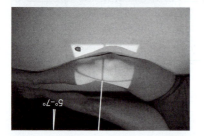
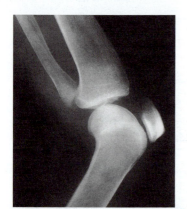

Manual Factors

Part Thickness (cm)	mA	kVp	Time	mAs	SID	Image Receptor Size	CR, DR Exposure Indicator	Grid	HF, 1Ø or 3Ø

AEC Factors

Part Thickness (cm)	mA	kVp	AEC Detector	mAs	Density Comp.	Image Receptor Size	CR, DR Exposure Indicator	Grid	HF, 1Ø or 3Ø

Notes: _____ Competency: ____/____/____

_____ Instructor: _____

Lower Extremity

Knee
AP oblique (lateral rotation)

Patient Position
• Position patient supine with affected knee extended.

Part Position
• Rotate affected extremity laterally until 45-degree rotation is achieved.
• Center knee to IR at level ½ inch (1.3 cm) below apex of patella.

Central Ray
• Direct ½ inch (1.3 cm) inferior to patellar apex.
• Angle varies as follows, depending on ASIS-to-tabletop measurement:

<19 cm	3 to 5 degrees (*caudad*)
19 to 24 cm	0 degrees
>24 cm	3 to 5 degrees (*cephalad*)

Collimation:
Adjust to 8 × 10 inch (18 × 24 cm). Adjust to 1 inch (2.5 cm) beyond the sides. Place side marker in the collimated exposure field.

kVp: 70 (non-grid), 85 (grid)   *Reference: 14th edition ATLAS p. 1:350.*

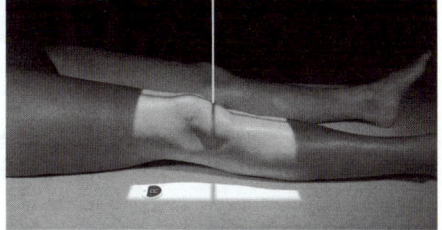

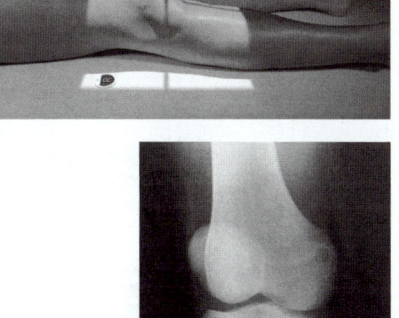

Manual Factors

Part Thickness (cm)	mA	kVp	Time	mAs	SID	Image Receptor Size	CR, DR Exposure Indicator	Grid	HF, 1Ø or 3Ø

AEC Factors

Part Thickness (cm)	mA	kVp	AEC Detector	mAs	Density Comp.	Image Receptor Size	CR, DR Exposure Indicator	Grid	HF, 1Ø or 3Ø

Notes: _____ Competency: _____/____/____

Instructor: _____

Lower Extremity

Knee
AP oblique (medial rotation)

Patient Position
- Position patient supine with affected knee extended.

Part Position
- Rotate extremity medially until 45-degree rotation is achieved.
- Center knee to IR at level ½ inch (1.3 cm) below apex of patella.

Central Ray
- Direct ½ inch (1.3 cm) inferior to patellar apex.
- Angle varies as follows, depending on ASIS-to-tabletop measurement:

<19 cm	3 to 5 degrees (*caudad*)
19 to 24 cm	0 degrees
>24 cm	3 to 5 degrees (*cephalad*)

Collimation:
Adjust to 8 × 10 inch (18 × 24 cm) on the collimator. Adjust to 1 inch (2.5 cm) beyond the sides. Place side marker in the collimated exposure field.

kVp: 70 (non-grid), 85 (grid)   *Reference: 14th edition ATLAS p. 1:351.*

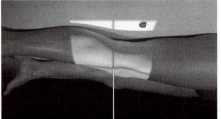
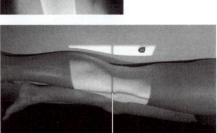

Manual Factors

Part Thickness (cm)	mA	kVp	Time	mAs	SID	Image Receptor Size	CR, DR Exposure Indicator	Grid	HF, 1Ø or 3Ø

AEC Factors

Part Thickness (cm)	mA	kVp	AEC Detector	mAs	Density Comp.	Image Receptor Size	CR, DR Exposure Indicator	Grid	HF, 1Ø or 3Ø

Notes: _____ Competency: ____/____/____

_____ Instructor: _____

Lower Extremity

Intercondylar Fossa
PA axial   HOLMBLAD METHOD*

Patient Position
• Have patient kneel on radiographic table with affected knee in contact with IR.

Part Position
• Center knee to IR by placing at level of patellar apex.
• Flex knee 70 degrees from full extension.

Central Ray
• Perpendicular to long axis of lower leg, entering midpoint of IR.

Collimation:
Adjust to 8 × 10 inches (18 × 24 cm). Adjust to 1 inch (2.5 cm) beyond the sides. Place side marker in the collimated exposure field.

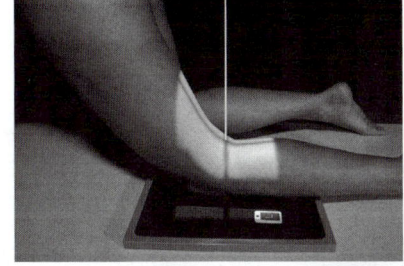

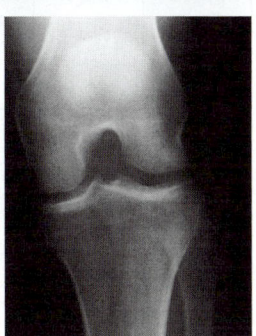

kVp: 70

*See ATLAS for alternate body positions.
Reference: 14th edition ATLAS p. 1:352.*

Manual Factors

Part Thickness (cm)	mA	kVp	Time	mAs	SID	Image Receptor Size	CR, DR Exposure Indicator	Grid	HF, 1Ø or 3Ø

AEC Factors

Part Thickness (cm)	mA	kVp	AEC Detector	mAs	Density Comp.	Image Receptor Size	CR, DR Exposure Indicator	Grid	HF, 1Ø or 3Ø

Notes: _____ Competency: ____/____/____

_____ Instructor: _____

Lower Extremity

Intercondylar Fossa
PA axial   **CAMP-COVENTRY METHOD**

Patient Position
• Position patient prone with hips equidistant from table.

Part Position
• Flex affected knee 40 to 50 degrees, and rest on suitable support.
• Adjust leg so that no medial or lateral rotation occurs.

Central Ray
• Perpendicular to long axis of leg, entering knee joint at popliteal depression (with central ray angled 40 to 50 degrees from vertical).

Collimation:
Adjust to 8 × 10 inches (18 × 24 cm). Adjust to 1 inch (2.5 cm) beyond the sides. Place side marker in the collimated exposure field.

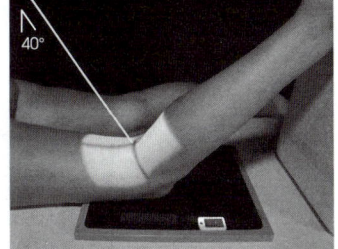

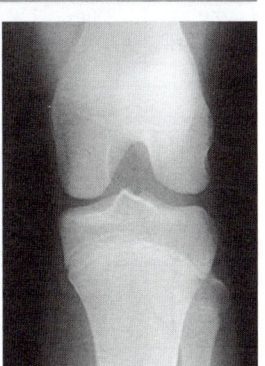

kVp: 70

Reference: 14th edition ATLAS p. 1:354.

Manual Factors

Part Thickness (cm)	mA	kVp	Time	mAs	SID	Image Receptor Size	CR, DR Exposure Indicator	Grid	HF, 1Ø or 3Ø

AEC Factors

Part Thickness (cm)	mA	kVp	AEC Detector	mAs	Density Comp.	Image Receptor Size	CR, DR Exposure Indicator	Grid	HF, 1Ø or 3Ø

Notes: _____ Competency: _____/_____/_____

_____ Instructor: _____

Lower Extremity

Patella
PA

Patient Position
• Position patient prone with knee extended.

Part Position
• Center patella and adjust leg to be parallel to IR plane.
• Heel is typically rotated 5 to 10 degrees laterally.

Central Ray
• Perpendicular, entering midpopliteal area.

Collimation:
Adjust to 6 × 6 inches (15 × 15 cm). Place side marker in the collimated exposure field.

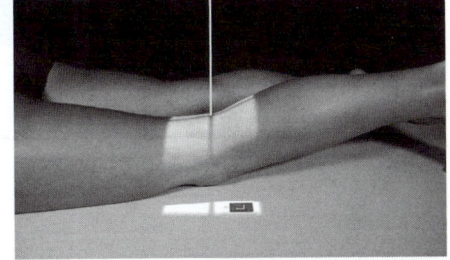

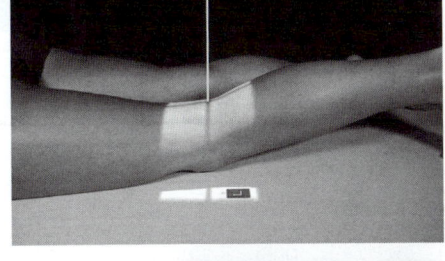

kVp: 85 (grid)

Reference: 14th edition ATLAS p. 1:357.

Manual Factors

Part Thickness (cm)	mA	kVp	Time	mAs	SID	Image Receptor Size	CR, DR Exposure Indicator	Grid	HF, 1Ø or 3Ø

AEC Factors

Part Thickness (cm)	mA	kVp	AEC Detector	mAs	Density Comp.	Image Receptor Size	CR, DR Exposure Indicator	Grid	HF, 1Ø or 3Ø

Notes: _____ Competency: ____/____/____

Instructor: _____

Lower Extremity

Patella
Lateral (mediolateral)

Patient Position
- Position patient on affected side.

Part Position
- Adjust affected knee to be flexed 5 to 10 degrees.
- Center IR to patella.
- Adjust body rotation so that patella is perpendicular to IR.

Central Ray
- Perpendicular to IR, entering knee at midpatellofemoral joint.
- Collimate to patella.

Collimation:
Adjust to 4 × 4 inches (10 × 10 cm). Place side marker in the collimated exposure field.

kVp: 85 (grid)

Reference: 14th edition ATLAS p. 1:358.

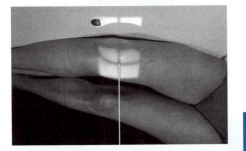
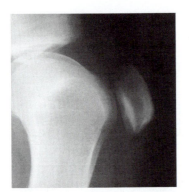

Manual Factors

Part Thickness (cm)	mA	kVp	Time	mAs	SID	Image Receptor Size	CR, DR Exposure Indicator	Grid	HF, 1Ø or 3Ø

AEC Factors

Part Thickness (cm)	mA	kVp	AEC Detector	mAs	Density Comp.	Image Receptor Size	CR, DR Exposure Indicator	Grid	HF, 1Ø or 3Ø

Notes: _____ Competency: _____/____/____

_____ Instructor: _____

Lower Extremity

Patella
Tangential SETTEGAST METHOD

Patient Position
• Position patient prone with foot resting on table.

Part Position
• Have patient flex affected knee slowly until patella is perpendicular to IR, if condition permits.
• Adjust leg so that no rotation occurs, and immobilize.

Central Ray
• Perpendicular to joint space between patella and femur if patella is perpendicular.
• If patella is not perpendicular, angulation depends on degree of flexion of knee, usually 15 to 20 degrees.

Collimation:
Adjust to 4 × 4 inches (10 × 10 cm). Place side marker in the collimated exposure field.

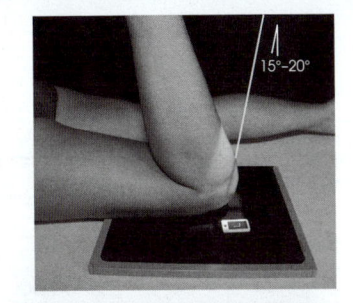

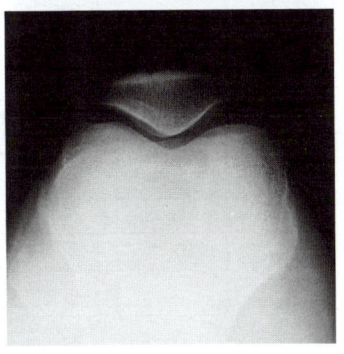

kVp: 70   *Reference: 14th edition ATLAS p. 1:362.*

Manual Factors

Part Thickness (cm)	mA	kVp	Time	mAs	SID	Image Receptor Size	CR, DR Exposure Indicator	Grid	HF, 1Ø or 3Ø

AEC Factors

Part Thickness (cm)	mA	kVp	AEC Detector	mAs	Density Comp.	Image Receptor Size	CR, DR Exposure Indicator	Grid	HF, 1Ø or 3Ø

Notes: _____ Competency: ____/____/____

Instructor: _____

Lower Extremity

Femur
AP*

Patient Position
- Position patient supine with toes up.
- Adjust pelvis to place ASIS equidistant from table.

Part Position
- Center affected femur to midline of grid.
- Image distal femur by placing bottom of IR 2 inches (5 cm) below knee joint.
- Rotate extremity internally to place it in true anatomic position.
- Apply gonad shielding.

Central Ray
- Perpendicular to midfemur and center of IR.

Collimation:
1 inch (2.5 cm) on sides of shadow of thigh and 17 inches (43 cm) in length. Place side marker in the collimated exposure field.

kVp: 85

*See ATLAS p. 1:364 for proximal femur instructions.
Reference: 14th edition ATLAS p. 1:364.

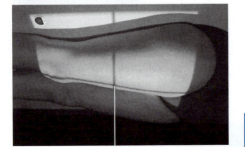
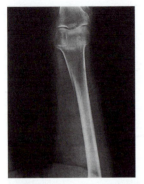

Manual Factors

Part Thickness (cm)	mA	kVp	Time	mAs	SID	Image Receptor Size	CR, DR Exposure Indicator	Grid	HF, 1Ø or 3Ø

AEC Factors

Part Thickness (cm)	mA	kVp	AEC Detector	mAs	Density Comp.	Image Receptor Size	CR, DR Exposure Indicator	Grid	HF, 1Ø or 3Ø

Notes: _____ Competency: ___/___/___

_____ Instructor: _____

Lower Extremity

Femur
Lateral*

Patient Position
• Position patient on affected side, with knee flexed about 45 degrees.

Part Position
• Center affected femur to midline of grid.
• Image distal femur by drawing uppermost extremity forward and supporting it at hip level.
• Adjust femur so that epicondyles are perpendicular to tabletop.
• Place bottom of IR 2 inches (5 cm) below knee joint.
• Apply gonad shielding.

Central Ray
• Perpendicular to midfemur.

Collimation:
1 inch (2.5 cm) on sides of shadow of thigh and 17 inches (43 cm) in length. Place side marker in the collimated exposure field.

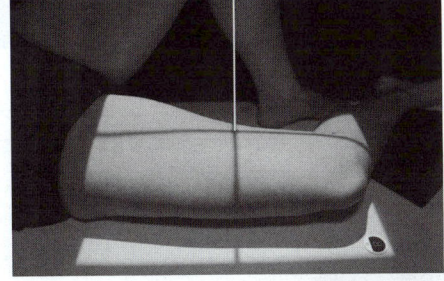

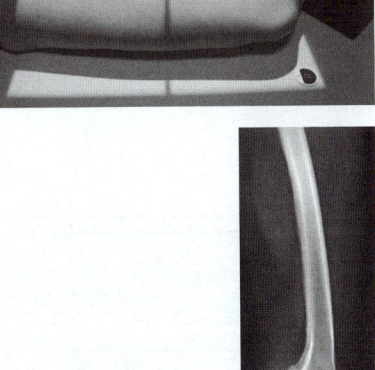

kVp: 85

See ATLAS p. 1:366 for proximal femur instructions.
Reference: 14th edition ATLAS p. 1:366.

Manual Factors

Part Thickness (cm)	mA	kVp	Time	mAs	SID	Image Receptor Size	CR, DR Exposure Indicator	Grid	HF, 1Ø or 3Ø

AEC Factors

Part Thickness (cm)	mA	kVp	AEC Detector	mAs	Density Comp.	Image Receptor Size	CR, DR Exposure Indicator	Grid	HF, 1Ø or 3Ø

Notes: _____ Competency: ____/____/____

Instructor: _____

Lower Extremity

Proximal Femora and Femoral Necks
AP oblique   MODIFIED CLEAVES METHOD

Patient Position
• Position patient supine.

Part Position
• Adjust pelvis so that no rotation occurs.
• Have patient flex hips and knees.
• Abduct thighs to approximately 45 degrees from vertical; brace soles of feet together.
• Shield gonads.

Respiration:
Suspend.

Central Ray
• Perpendicular, entering midline approximately 1 inch (2.5 cm) superior to symphysis pubis.
• Perpendicular to femoral neck for unilateral.

Collimation:
Adjust to 14 × 17 inches (35 × 43 cm). For smaller patients, collimate 1 inch (2.5 cm) beyond the skin shadow on the sides. Place side marker in the collimated exposure field.

NOTE: Adapt for unilateral examination by flexing and abducting affected extremity.

kVp: 85

Reference: 14th edition ATLAS p. 1-394

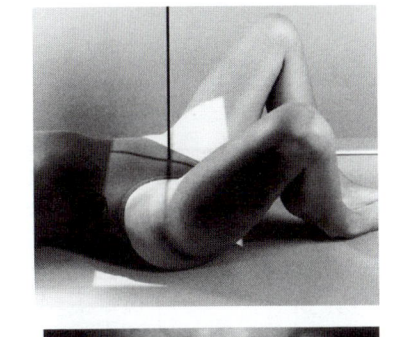

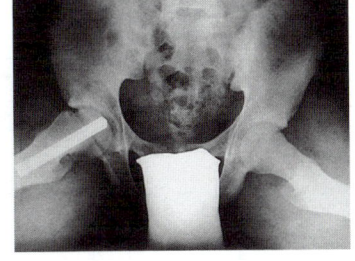

Manual Factors

Part Thickness (cm)	mA	kVp	Time	mAs	SID	Image Receptor Size	CR, DR Exposure Indicator	Grid	HF, 1Ø or 3Ø

AEC Factors

Part Thickness (cm)	mA	kVp	AEC Detector	mAs	Density Comp.	Image Receptor Size	CR, DR Exposure Indicator	Grid	HF, 1Ø or 3Ø

Notes: _____ Competency: _____/_____/_____

_____ Instructor: _____

Lower Extremity

Hip
AP

Patient Position
- Position patient supine.
- Adjust ASIS equidistant from table.

Part Position
- Rotate affected extremity 15 to 20 degrees medially; center hip to IR.
- Shield gonads.

Respiration:
Suspend.

Central Ray
- Perpendicular to point 2½ inches (6 cm) distal on line drawn perpendicular to midpoint of line between ASIS and pubic symphysis.

Collimation:
Adjust to 10 × 12 inches (24 × 30 cm). Place side marker in the collimated exposure field.

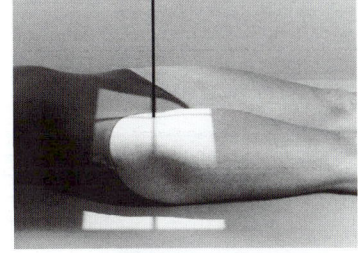

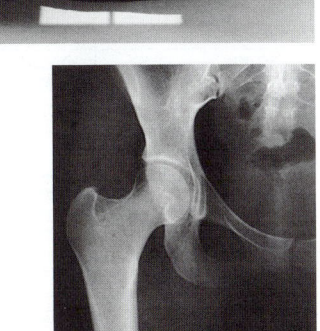

kVp: 85

Reference: 14th edition ATLAS p. 1:398.

Manual Factors									
Part Thickness (cm)	mA	kVp	Time	mAs	SID	Image Receptor Size	CR, DR Exposure Indicator	Grid	HF, 1Ø or 3Ø

AEC Factors									
Part Thickness (cm)	mA	kVp	AEC Detector	mAs	Density Comp.	Image Receptor Size	CR, DR Exposure Indicator	Grid	HF, 1Ø or 3Ø

Notes: _____ Competency: ____/____/____

Instructor: _____

Lower Extremity

Hip
Lateral LAUENSTEIN AND HICKEY METHODS

Patient Position
• Start with patient supine, and turn patient slightly toward affected side to posterior oblique body position.

Part Position
• Flex affected knee and hip and rest on table; center affected hip to midline of grid.
• Have patient extend unaffected knee.
• Shield gonads.

Respiration:
Suspend.

Central Ray
• Perpendicular to hip at point midway between ASIS and pubic symphysis for Lauenstein method and at cephalic angle of 20 to 25 degrees for Hickey method.

Collimation:
Adjust to 10 × 12 inches (24 × 30 cm). Place side marker in the collimated exposure field.

kVp: 85   *Reference: 14th edition ATLAS p. 1:400.*

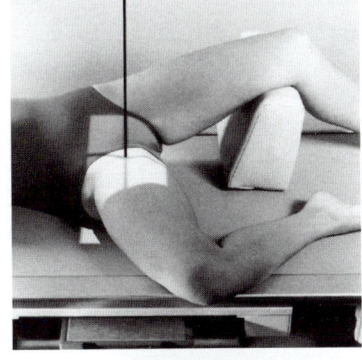
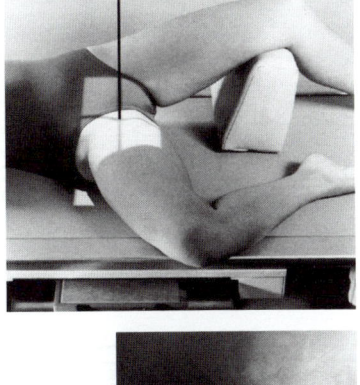

Manual Factors

Part Thickness (cm)	mA	kVp	Time	mAs	SID	Image Receptor Size	CR, DR Exposure Indicator	Grid	HF, 1Ø or 3Ø

AEC Factors

Part Thickness (cm)	mA	kVp	AEC Detector	mAs	Density Comp.	Image Receptor Size	CR, DR Exposure Indicator	Grid	HF, 1Ø or 3Ø

Notes: _____ Competency: _____/_____/_____

_____ Instructor: _____

Lower Extremity

Hip
Axiolateral DANELIUS-MILLER METHOD

Patient Position
• Position patient supine with level of greater trochanter elevated to center of IR.

Part Position
• Have patient flex knee and hip of unaffected side.
• Elevate patient's foot, and rest on suitable support.
• Adjust pelvis so that no rotation occurs.
• Rotate affected leg medially 15 to 20 degrees unless contraindicated.

Respiration:
Suspend.

Central Ray
• Perpendicular to long axis of femoral neck and IR.

Collimation:
Adjust to 10 × 12 inches (24 × 30 cm). Place side marker in the collimated exposure field.

▼ COMPENSATING FILTER
• Image is improved and can be performed with one projection if filter is used.

kVp: 90   *Reference: 14th edition ATLAS p. 1:402.*

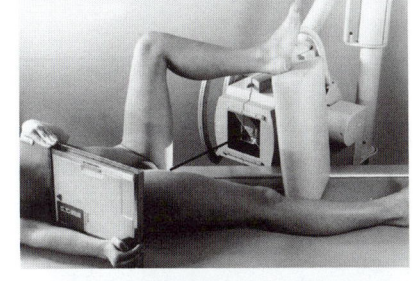

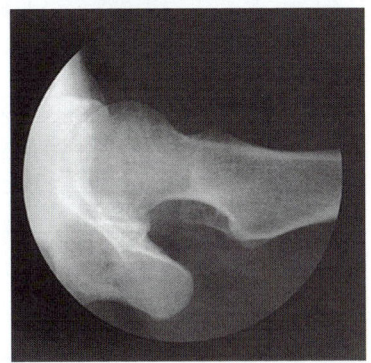

Manual Factors

Part Thickness (cm)	mA	kVp	Time	mAs	SID	Image Receptor Size	CR, DR Exposure Indicator	Grid	HF, 1Ø or 3Ø

AEC Factors

Part Thickness (cm)	mA	kVp	AEC Detector	mAs	Density Comp.	Image Receptor Size	CR, DR Exposure Indicator	Grid	HF, 1Ø or 3Ø

Notes: _____ Competency: _____/_____/_____

_____ Instructor: _____

Lower Extremity

Pelvis and Proximal Femora
AP

Patient Position
• Position patient supine.

Part Position
• Center midsagittal plane to grid; adjust so that ASIS are equidistant from table.
• Rotate feet and lower extremities medially 15 to 20 degrees unless contraindicated.
• Center IR approximately 2 inches (5 cm) superior to pubic symphysis and 2 inches (5 cm) inferior to ASIS.
• Use gonad shielding as appropriate.

Respiration:
Suspend.

Central Ray
• Perpendicular to midpoint of IR.

Collimation:
Adjust to 14 × 17 inches (35 × 43 cm). For smaller patients, collimate 1 inch (2.5 cm) beyond the skin shadow on the sides. Place side marker in the collimated exposure field.

kVp: 85   *Reference: 14th edition ATLAS p. 1:389.*

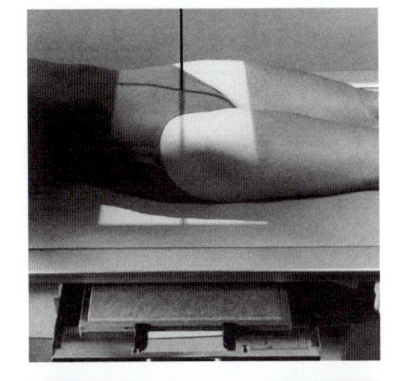

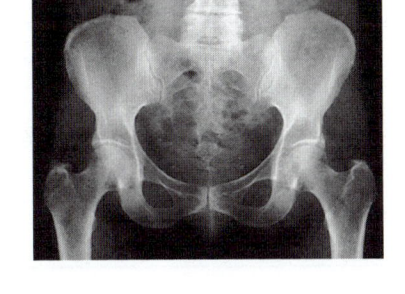

Manual Factors

Part Thickness (cm)	mA	kVp	Time	mAs	SID	Image Receptor Size	CR, DR Exposure Indicator	Grid	HF, 1Ø or 3Ø

AEC Factors

Part Thickness (cm)	mA	kVp	AEC Detector	mAs	Density Comp.	Image Receptor Size	CR, DR Exposure Indicator	Grid	HF, 1Ø or 3Ø

Notes: _____ Competency: _____/___/___

_____ Instructor: _____

Lower Extremity

Atlas and Axis:
  AP (open mouth), 138
Dens:
  AP; FUCHS METHOD, 140
Cervical Vertebrae:
  AP axial, 142
  Lateral; GRANDY METHOD, 144
  Flexion and extension lateral, 146
  AP axial oblique (RPO and LPO), 148
  PA axial oblique (RAO and LAO), 150
  Trauma lateral (dorsal decubitus), 152
  Trauma AP axial oblique, 154

Cervicothoracic Region:
  Lateral; SWIMMER'S TECHNIQUE, 156
Thoracic Vertebrae:
  AP, 158
  Lateral, 160
Lumbar-Lumbosacral Vertebrae:
  AP, 162
  Lateral, 164
L5-S1 Lumbosacral Junction:
  Lateral, 166
Lumbar Zygapophyseal Joints:
  AP oblique (RPO and LPO), 168
Lumbosacral Junction and Sacroiliac Joints:
  AP axial; FERGUSON METHOD, 170

Sacroiliac Joints:
  AP oblique (RPO and LPO), 172
Sacrum:
  AP axial, 174
  Lateral, 176
Coccyx:
  AP axial, 178
  Lateral, 180
Thoracolumbar Spine: Scoliosis
  AP, PA, or lateral; FERGUSON METHOD, 182

Vertebral Column

Atlas and Axis
AP (open mouth)

Patient Position
- Position patient upright or supine.

Part Position
- Center midsagittal plane to midline of table, arms at sides, shoulders in same plane.
- Center IR at level of axis.
- Open mouth wide; adjust head so that line from lower edge of upper incisors to mastoid process is perpendicular to IR.
- Shield gonads.

Respiration:
Have patient phonate "ah" during exposure.

Central Ray
- Perpendicular to center of IR, entering open mouth.

Collimation:
Adjust to 5 × 5 inches (13 × 13 cm). Place side marker in the collimated exposure field.

kVp: 85

Reference: 14th edition ATLAS p. 1:438.

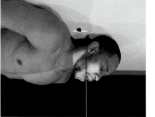
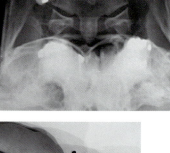

Manual Factors

Part Thickness (cm)	mA	kVp	Time	mAs	SID	Image Receptor Size	CR, DR Exposure Indicator	Grid	HF, 1Ø or 3Ø

AEC Factors

Part Thickness (cm)	mA	kVp	AEC Detector	mAs	Density Comp.	Image Receptor Size	CR, DR Exposure Indicator	Grid	HF, 1Ø or 3Ø

Notes: _____ Competency: _____/____/____

_____ Instructor: _____

Vertebral Column

Dens
AP FUCHS METHOD

Patient Position
- Position patient supine.

Part Position
- Adjust head so that midsagittal plane is perpendicular to IR.
- Extend chin until a line between chin and tip of mastoid process is perpendicular to IR.
- Center IR to level of tips of mastoid process.
- Shield gonads.

Respiration:
Suspend.

Central Ray
- Perpendicular to center of IR, entering midsagittal plane just distal to tip of chin.

Collimation:
Adjust to 5 × 5 inches (13 × 13 cm). Place side marker in the collimated exposure field.

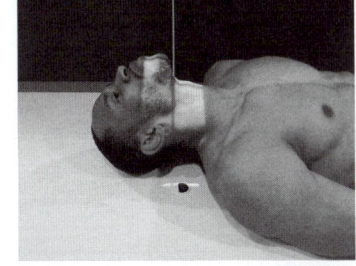

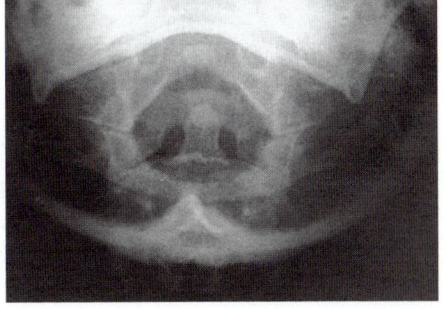

kVp: 85

Reference: 14th edition ATLAS p. 1:437.

Manual Factors									
Part Thickness (cm)	mA	kVp	Time	mAs	SID	Image Receptor Size	CR, DR Exposure Indicator	Grid	HF, 1Ø or 3Ø

AEC Factors									
Part Thickness (cm)	mA	kVp	AEC Detector	mAs	Density Comp.	Image Receptor Size	CR, DR Exposure Indicator	Grid	HF, 1Ø or 3Ø

Notes: _____ Competency: _____/_____/_____

Instructor: _____

Vertebral Column

Cervical Vertebrae
AP axial

Patient Position
• Position patient upright or supine.

Part Position
• Center midsagittal plane to IR.
• Have patient place arms at sides.
• Center IR at level of C4, and adjust a line between upper occlusal plane and mastoid tip perpendicular to IR.
• Shield gonads.

Respiration:
Suspend.

Central Ray
• Angle 15 to 20 degrees cephalad, entering slightly inferior to thyroid cartilage and exiting C4.

Collimation:
Adjust 10 inches (24 cm) lengthwise and 1 inch (2.5 cm) beyond skin shadow on sides. Place side marker in the collimated exposure field.

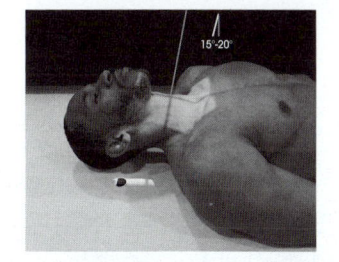

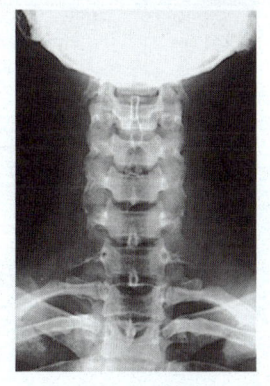

kVp: 85

Reference: 14th edition ATLAS p. 1:441.

Manual Factors

Part Thickness (cm)	mA	kVp	Time	mAs	SID	Image Receptor Size	CR, DR Exposure Indicator	Grid	HF, 1Ø or 3Ø

AEC Factors

Part Thickness (cm)	mA	kVp	AEC Detector	mAs	Density Comp.	Image Receptor Size	CR, DR Exposure Indicator	Grid	HF, 1Ø or 3Ø

Notes: _____ Competency: _____/_____/_____

_____ Instructor: _____

Vertebral Column

Cervical Vertebrae
Lateral GRANDY METHOD

Patient Position
- Position patient seated or standing in lateral position.

Part Position
- Center coronal plane through mastoid processes to IR.
- Adjust shoulders to same horizontal level and body to true lateral position
- Have patient elevate chin slightly and relax shoulders. If necessary, attach weights to wrists to help lower shoulders.
- Shield gonads.

Respiration:
Suspend.

Central Ray
- Horizontal and perpendicular to IR, entering C4.
- SID of 72 inches (180 cm) is recommended.

Collimation:
Adjust to 10 × 12 inches (24 × 30 cm). Place side marker in the collimated exposure field.

kVp: 85

Reference: 14th edition ATLAS p. 1:443.

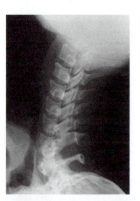
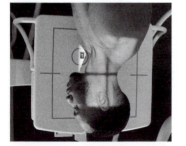

Manual Factors									
Part Thickness (cm)	mA	kVp	Time	mAs	SID	Image Receptor Size	CR, DR Exposure Indicator	Grid	HF, 1Ø or 3Ø

AEC Factors									
Part Thickness (cm)	mA	kVp	AEC Detector	mAs	Density Comp.	Image Receptor Size	CR, DR Exposure Indicator	Grid	HF, 1Ø or 3Ø

Notes: _____ Competency: ____/____/____

_____ Instructor: _____

Vertebral Column

Cervical Vertebrae
Flexion and extension lateral

Patient Position
- Position patient seated or standing in lateral position.

Part Position
- Center spine to IR.
- Keep midsagittal plane of head and neck parallel to plane of IR and ask patient to do the following: (1) Drop head forward and draw chin as close as possible to chest to place cervical vertebrae in full flexion—expose—and (2) elevate chin as much as possible to place cervical vertebrae in full extension.
- Shield gonads.

Respiration:
Suspend.

Central Ray
- Horizontal and perpendicular to IR, entering C4.
- SID of 72 inches (180 cm) is recommended.

Collimation:
Adjust to 10 × 12 inches (24 × 30 cm). Place side marker in the collimated exposure field.

kVp: 85

Reference: 14th edition ATLAS p. 1:445.

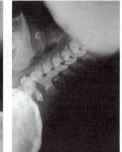

Manual Factors

Part Thickness (cm)	mA	kVp	Time	mAs	SID	Image Receptor Size	CR, DR Exposure Indicator	Grid	HF, 1Ø or 3Ø

AEC Factors

Part Thickness (cm)	mA	kVp	AEC Detector	mAs	Density Comp.	Image Receptor Size	CR, DR Exposure Indicator	Grid	HF, 1Ø or 3Ø

Notes: _____ Competency: ____/____/____

_____ Instructor: _____

Vertebral Column

Cervical Vertebrae
AP axial oblique (RPO and LPO)

Patient Position
• Position patient seated or standing.

Part Position
• Rotate body to 45 degrees, with side of interest farther from IR.
• Have patient extend chin slightly while looking forward.
• Center spine to IR.
• Center IR to C3.
• Shield gonads.
• Take both oblique projections.

Respiration:
Suspend.

Central Ray
• Angle 15 to 20 degrees cephalad, entering C4.
• SID of 60 to 72 inches (152 to 183 cm) is recommended.

Collimation:
Adjust to 10 × 12 inch (24 × 30 cm). Place side marker in the
collimated exposure field.

kVp: 85   *Reference: 14th edition ATLAS p. 1:447.*

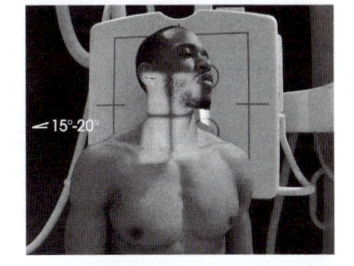

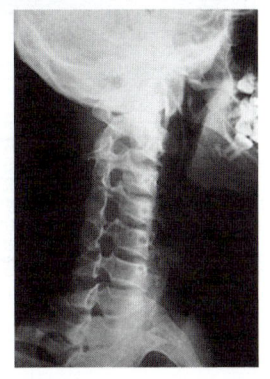

Manual Factors									
Part Thickness (cm)	mA	kVp	Time	mAs	SID	Image Receptor Size	CR, DR Exposure Indicator	Grid	HF, 1Ø or 3Ø

AEC Factors									
Part Thickness (cm)	mA	kVp	AEC Detector	mAs	Density Comp.	Image Receptor Size	CR, DR Exposure Indicator	Grid	HF, 1Ø or 3Ø

Notes: _____

Competency: ____/____/____

Instructor: _____

Vertebral Column

Cervical Vertebrae
PA axial oblique (RAO and LAO)

Patient Position
• Position patient upright or prone.

Part Position
• Rotate body 45 degrees with side of interest closer to IR.
• Extend chin slightly.
• Center spine to IR.
• Center IR to C5.
• Shield gonads.
• Take both oblique projections.

Respiration:
Suspend.

Central Ray
• Angle 15 to 20 degrees caudad, entering C4.
• SID of 60 to 72 inches (150 to 180 cm) is recommended.

Collimation:
Adjust to 10 × 12 inch (24 × 30 cm). Place side marker in the collimated exposure field.

kVp: 85

Reference: 14th edition ATLAS p. 1:449.

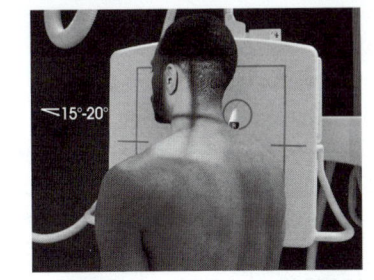

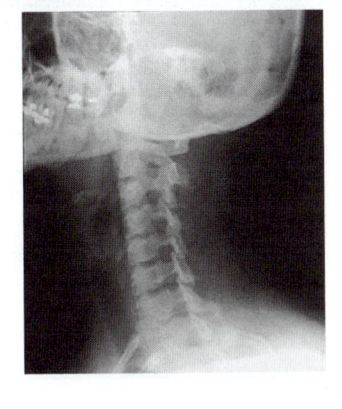

Manual Factors									
Part Thickness (cm)	mA	kVp	Time	mAs	SID	Image Receptor Size	CR, DR Exposure Indicator	Grid	HF, 1Ø or 3Ø

AEC Factors									
Part Thickness (cm)	mA	kVp	AEC Detector	mAs	Density Comp.	Image Receptor Size	CR, DR Exposure Indicator	Grid	HF, 1Ø or 3Ø

Notes: _____ Competency: _____/___/___

_____ Instructor: _____

Vertebral Column

Cervical Vertebrae
Trauma lateral (dorsal decubitus)

Patient Position
- Position patient supine.
- Do not move patient or remove cervical collar without consulting physician.

Part Position
- Place IR next to patient's shoulder, and center at level of C4.
- Do not rotate or extend neck.
- Depress shoulders as much as possible. If necessary, loop a bandage around patient's feet and affix to wrists so that extending knees depresses shoulders.
- Shield gonads.

Respiration:
Suspend.

Central Ray
- Angle horizontal and perpendicular, entering C4.
- SID of 60 to 72 inches (150 to 180 cm) is recommended.

Collimation:
Adjust to 10 × 12 inch (24 × 30 cm). Place side marker in the collimated exposure field.

kVp: 85 (grid)

Reference: 14th edition ATLAS p. 2:124.

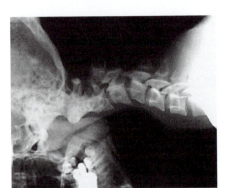
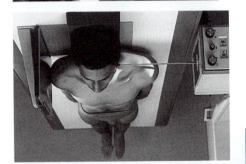

Manual Factors

Part Thickness (cm)	mA	kVp	Time	mAs	SID	Image Receptor Size	CR, DR Exposure Indicator	Grid	HF, 1Ø or 3Ø

AEC Factors

Part Thickness (cm)	mA	kVp	AEC Detector	mAs	Density Comp.	Image Receptor Size	CR, DR Exposure Indicator	Grid	HF, 1Ø or 3Ø

Notes: _____ Competency: _____/_____/_____

_____ Instructor: _____

Vertebral Column

Cervical Vertebrae
Trauma AP axial oblique

Patient Position
- Position patient supine.
- Do not move patient or remove cervical collar without consulting physician.

Part Position
- Brace head and neck and lift only enough to slide IR under neck.
- Place IR under backboard if patient is on backboard.
- Center IR to mastoid on side opposite x-ray tube. (This allows angled central ray to project image of side of interest in center of image.)
- Shield gonads.

Central Ray
- Adjust 45 degrees medial and 15 to 20 degrees cephalad, entering level of C4.

Collimation:
Adjust to 10 × 12 inch (24 × 30 cm). Place side marker in the collimated exposure field.

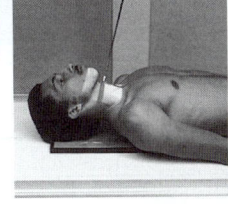
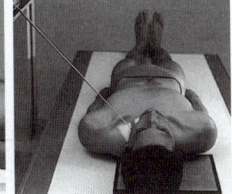
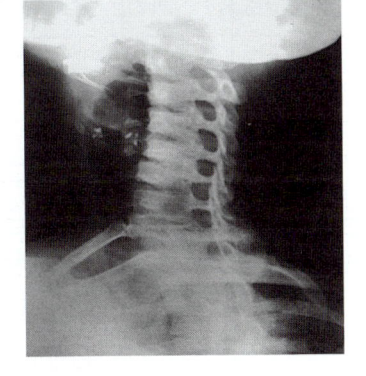

kVp: 75

Reference: 14th edition ATLAS p. 2:127.

Manual Factors

Part Thickness (cm)	mA	kVp	Time	mAs	SID	Image Receptor Size	CR, DR Exposure Indicator	Grid	HF, 1Ø or 3Ø

AEC Factors

Part Thickness (cm)	mA	kVp	AEC Detector	mAs	Density Comp.	Image Receptor Size	CR, DR Exposure Indicator	Grid	HF, 1Ø or 3Ø

Notes: _____ Competency: ____/____/____

Instructor: _____

Vertebral Column

Cervicothoracic Region
Lateral   SWIMMER'S TECHNIQUE

Patient Position
- Position patient seated, standing, or in lateral recumbent position.

Part Position
- Center midcoronal plane to IR.
- Elevate arm adjacent to vertical IR holder, and rest it on head.
- Rotate this shoulder forward or backward according to patient's condition. Rotate opposite shoulder in opposite direction.
- Adjust head and body so that midsagittal plane is parallel to IR.
- Shield gonads.

Respiration:
Suspend.

Central Ray
- Perpendicular to C7-T1 interspace.
- Use 5-degree caudal angulation if shoulder farthest from IR cannot be adequately depressed.

Collimation:
Adjust to 10 × 12 inches (24 × 30 cm). Place side marker in the collimated exposure field.

COMPENSATING FILTER
- Use of a specially designed compensating filter will improve image quality.

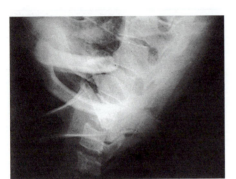

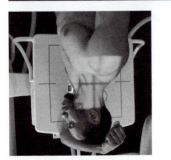

Manual Factors

Part Thickness (cm)	mA	kVp	Time	mAs	SID	Image Receptor Size	CR, DR Exposure Indicator	Grid	HF, 1Ø or 3Ø

AEC Factors

Part Thickness (cm)	mA	kVp	AEC Detector	mAs	Density Comp.	Image Receptor Size	CR, DR Exposure Indicator	Grid	HF, 1Ø or 3Ø

Notes: _____ Competency: _____/____/____

_____ Instructor: _____

Vertebral Column

Thoracic Vertebrae
AP

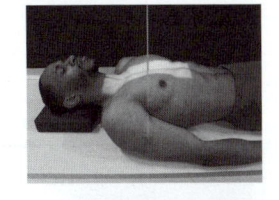

Patient Position
- Position patient supine or upright. If possible, orient the patient so the lower thorax is at the cathode end of the x-ray tube.

Part Position
- Center midsagittal plane to IR.
- Position top of IR 1½ to 2 inches (3.8 to 5 cm) above shoulders.
- Have patient hold arms at sides, shoulders in same plane.
- Flex hips and knees to reduce dorsal kyphosis if patient is supine.
- Shield gonads.

Respiration:
Suspended at end of full expiration.

Central Ray
- Perpendicular to IR. The central ray should be approximately midway between jugular notch and xiphoid process.

Collimation:
Adjust to 7 × 17 inches (18 × 43 cm). Place side marker in the collimated exposure field.

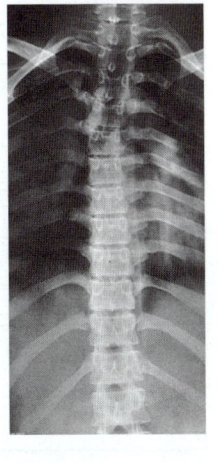

◣ COMPENSATING FILTER
- Use of specially designed compensating filter will improve image quality.

kVp: 90   *Reference: 14th edition ATLAS p. 1:458.*

Manual Factors

Part Thickness (cm)	mA	kVp	Time	mAs	SID	Image Receptor Size	CR, DR Exposure Indicator	Grid	HF, 1Ø or 3Ø

AEC Factors

Part Thickness (cm)	mA	kVp	AEC Detector	mAs	Density Comp.	Image Receptor Size	CR, DR Exposure Indicator	Grid	HF, 1Ø or 3Ø

Notes: _____ Competency: ____/____/____

Instructor: _____

Vertebral Column

Thoracic Vertebrae
Lateral

Patient Position
• Position patient in lateral recumbent position or upright.

Part Position
• Center posterior half of thorax to midline of grid.
• Place top of IR 1½ to 2 inches (3.8 to 5 cm) above relaxed shoulders.
• Elevate head to spine level. Extend arms forward.
• Place radiolucent support under lower thoracic region until spine is horizontal to tabletop.
• Shield gonads.

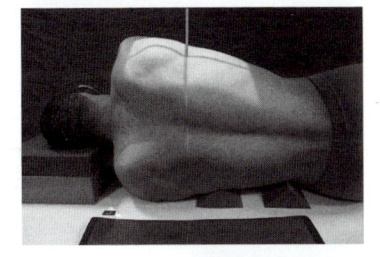

Respiration:
The exposure can be made while the patient continues to breath normally, the "breathing technique," to blur the pulmonary vascular markings and ribs or after breathing is suspended at the end of expiration.

Central Ray
• Perpendicular to center of IR at level of T7. Central ray enters posterior half of thorax.

Collimation:
Adjust to 7 × 17 inches (18 × 43 cm). Place side marker in the collimated exposure field.

kVp: 90   *Reference: 14th edition ATLAS p. 1:461.*

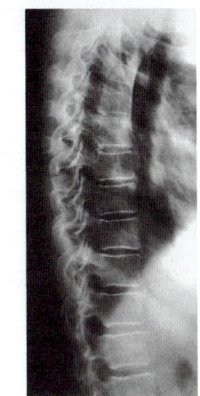

Manual Factors

Part Thickness (cm)	mA	kVp	Time	mAs	SID	Image Receptor Size	CR, DR Exposure Indicator	Grid	HF, 1Ø or 3Ø

AEC Factors

Part Thickness (cm)	mA	kVp	AEC Detector	mAs	Density Comp.	Image Receptor Size	CR, DR Exposure Indicator	Grid	HF, 1Ø or 3Ø

Notes: _____ Competency: _____/____/____

Instructor: _____

Vertebral Column

Lumbar-Lumbosacral Vertebrae
AP

Patient Position
• Position patient supine.

Part Position
• Center midsagittal plane to grid.
• Flex knees and hips enough to place back in firm contact with table.
• Center IR at iliac crests (L4).
• Shield gonads.

Respiration:
Suspend at the end of expiration.

Central Ray
• Perpendicular to center of IR, entering at level of iliac crests

Collimation:
Adjust to 8 × 17 inches (18 × 43 cm). Place side marker in the collimated exposure field.

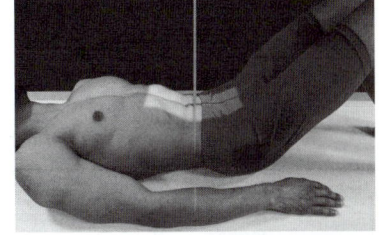

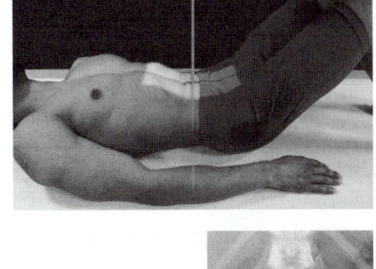

kVp: 90   *Reference: 14th edition ATLAS p. 1:467.*

Manual Factors

Part Thickness (cm)	mA	kVp	Time	mAs	SID	Image Receptor Size	CR, DR Exposure Indicator	Grid	HF, 1Ø or 3Ø

AEC Factors

Part Thickness (cm)	mA	kVp	AEC Detector	mAs	Density Comp.	Image Receptor Size	CR, DR Exposure Indicator	Grid	HF, 1Ø or 3Ø

Notes: _____ Competency: ____/____/____

Instructor: _____

Vertebral Column

Lumbar-Lumbosacral Vertebrae
Lateral

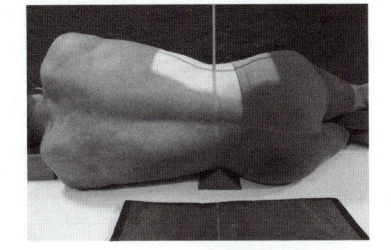

Patient Position
• Position patient lateral, with hips and knees flexed.

Part Position
• Center IR to level of iliac crests.
• Center midcoronal plane of body to grid.
• Extend arms forward.
• Place radiolucent support under lower thorax; adjust spine parallel to table.
• Place lead rubber behind patient to absorb radiation.
• Shield gonads.

Respiration:
Suspend at the end of expiration.

Central Ray
• Perpendicular to IR, entering midcoronal plane at level of iliac crests.

Collimation:
Adjust to 8 × 17 inches (18 × 43 cm). Place side marker in the collimated exposure field.

kVp: 96   *Reference: 14th edition ATLAS p. 1:471.*

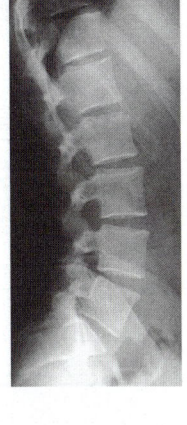

Manual Factors

Part Thickness (cm)	mA	kVp	Time	mAs	SID	Image Receptor Size	CR, DR Exposure Indicator	Grid	HF, 1Ø or 3Ø

AEC Factors

Part Thickness (cm)	mA	kVp	AEC Detector	mAs	Density Comp.	Image Receptor Size	CR, DR Exposure Indicator	Grid	HF, 1Ø or 3Ø

Notes: _____ Competency: _____/_____/_____

Instructor: _____

Vertebral Column

L5-S1 Lumbosacral Junction
Lateral

Patient Position
• Position patient lateral, with hips and knees extended or slightly flexed.

Part Position
• Extend arms forward.
• Place radiolucent support under lower thorax; adjust spine parallel to table.
• Adjust the midcoronal plane of the body (passing through the hips and shoulders) so that it is perpendicular to the IR.
• Shield gonads.

Respiration:
Suspend.

Central Ray
• On coronal plane 2 inches (5 cm) posterior to ASIS and 1½ inches inferior to crest.
• Have central ray parallel to interiliac line; caudal or cephalic angulation of 5 to 8 degrees may be required.

Collimation:
Adjust to 6 × 8 inches (15 × 20 cm). Place side marker in the collimated exposure field.

kVp: 96   *Reference: 14th edition ATLAS p. 1:473.*

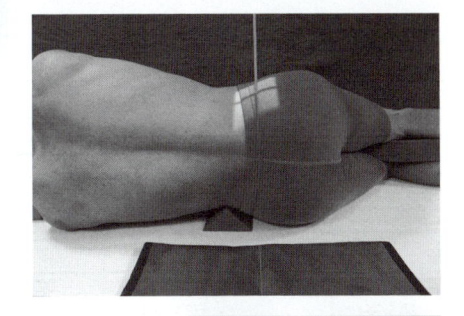

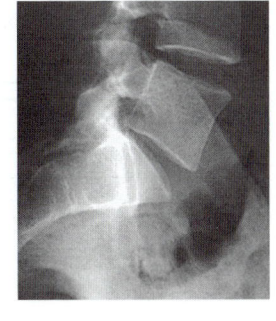

Manual Factors

Part Thickness (cm)	mA	kVp	Time	mAs	SID	Image Receptor Size	CR, DR Exposure Indicator	Grid	HF, 1Ø or 3Ø

AEC Factors

Part Thickness (cm)	mA	kVp	AEC Detector	mAs	Density Comp.	Image Receptor Size	CR, DR Exposure Indicator	Grid	HF, 1Ø or 3Ø

Notes: _____ Competency: ____/____/____

_____ Instructor: _____

Vertebral Column

Lumbar Zygapophyseal Joints
AP oblique (RPO and LPO)

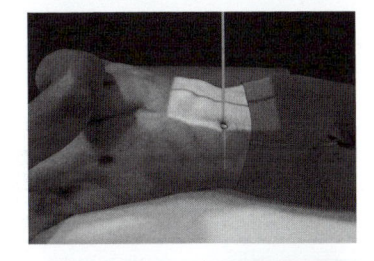

Patient Position
- Position patient posterior oblique, with side of interest closer to IR.

Part Position
- Adjust and support body obliquity to 45 degrees.
- Have patient place arms in a comfortable position, and center spine to midline of grid.
- Shield gonads.
- Take both oblique projections.

Respiration:
Suspend at end of expiration.

Central Ray
- Perpendicular, entering 2 inches (5 cm) medial to elevated ASIS and 1½ inches (3.8 cm) above iliac crest (L3).
- Center IR to central ray.

Collimation:
Adjust to 9 × 14 inches (23 × 35 cm). Place side marker in the collimated exposure field.

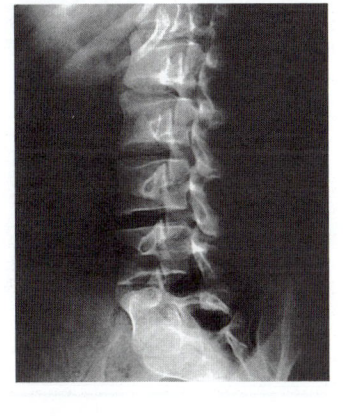

kVp: 90   *Reference: 14th edition ATLAS p. 1:475.*

Manual Factors

Part Thickness (cm)	mA	kVp	Time	mAs	SID	Image Receptor Size	CR, DR Exposure Indicator	Grid	HF, 1Ø or 3Ø

AEC Factors

Part Thickness (cm)	mA	kVp	AEC Detector	mAs	Density Comp.	Image Receptor Size	CR, DR Exposure Indicator	Grid	HF, 1Ø or 3Ø

Notes: _____ Competency: ____/____/____

Instructor: _____

Vertebral Column

Lumbosacral Junction and Sacroiliac Joints
AP axial FERGUSON METHOD

Patient Position
• Position patient supine, lower limbs extended.

Part Position
• Center midsagittal plane to grid.
• Extend lower limbs or flex hips and abduct to remove from path of central ray.
• Shield gonads.

Respiration:
Suspend.

Central Ray
• Angle 30 to 35 degrees cephalad through lumbosacral joint so that central ray enters about 1½ inches (3.8 cm) superior to pubic symphysis.
• Center IR to central ray.

Collimation:
Adjust to 8 × 10 inches (18 × 24 cm). Place side marker in the collimated exposure field.

kVp: 90   *Reference: 14th edition ATLAS p. 1:479.*

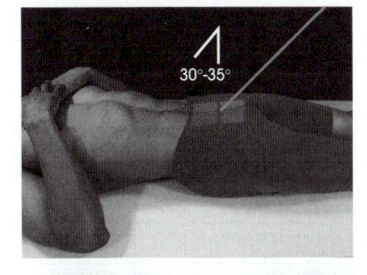

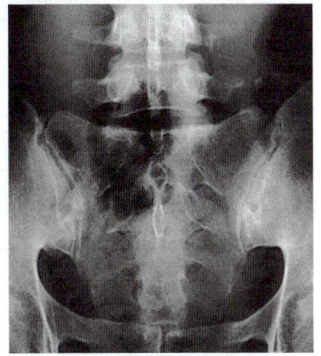

Manual Factors

Part Thickness (cm)	mA	kVp	Time	mAs	SID	Image Receptor Size	CR, DR Exposure Indicator	Grid	HF, 1Ø or 3Ø

AEC Factors

Part Thickness (cm)	mA	kVp	AEC Detector	mAs	Density Comp.	Image Receptor Size	CR, DR Exposure Indicator	Grid	HF, 1Ø or 3Ø

Notes: _____ Competency: _____/___/___

Instructor: _____

Vertebral Column

Sacroiliac Joints
AP oblique (RPO and LPO)

Patient Position
• Position patient supine.

Part Position
• Elevate and support side of interest 25 to 30 degrees from table.
• Align sagittal plane, passing 1 inch (2.5 cm) medial to elevated ASIS, and center to grid.
• Center IR at level of ASIS.
• Shield gonads.
• Take both oblique projections.

Respiration:
Suspend.

Central Ray
• Perpendicular to IR, entering 1 inch (2.5 cm) medial to elevated ASIS.

Collimation:
Adjust to 6 × 10 inches (15 × 24 cm). Place side marker in the collimated exposure field.

kVp: 90

Reference: 14th edition ATLAS p. 1:481.

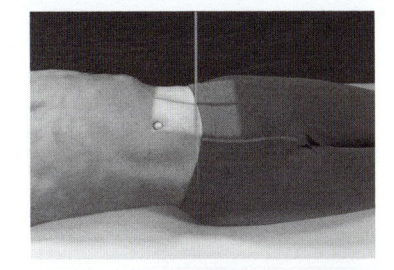

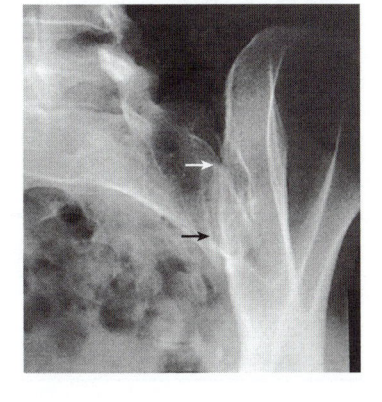

Manual Factors									
Part Thickness (cm)	mA	kVp	Time	mAs	SID	Image Receptor Size	CR, DR Exposure Indicator	Grid	HF, 1Ø or 3Ø

AEC Factors									
Part Thickness (cm)	mA	kVp	AEC Detector	mAs	Density Comp.	Image Receptor Size	CR, DR Exposure Indicator	Grid	HF, 1Ø or 3Ø

Notes: _____ Competency: _____/____/____

_____ Instructor: _____

Vertebral Column

Sacrum
AP axial

Patient Position
- Position patient supine.

Part Position
- Center midsagittal plane to center of grid.

Respiration:
Suspend.

Central Ray
- Angle 15 degrees cephalad and center on point 2 inches (5 cm) superior to pubic symphysis.
- Center IR to central ray.

Collimation:
Adjust to 8 × 10 inches (18 × 24 cm). Place side marker in the collimated exposure field.

kVp: 90

Reference: 14th edition ATLAS p. 1:485.

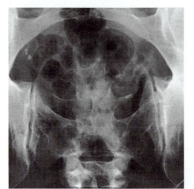

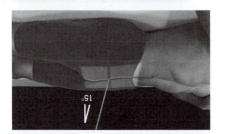

Manual Factors

Part Thickness (cm)	mA	kVp	Time	mAs	SID	Image Receptor Size	CR, DR Exposure Indicator	Grid	HF, 1Ø or 3Ø

AEC Factors

Part Thickness (cm)	mA	kVp	AEC Detector	mAs	Density Comp.	Image Receptor Size	CR, DR Exposure Indicator	Grid	HF, 1Ø or 3Ø

Notes: _____ Competency: _____/_____/_____

Instructor: _____

Vertebral Column

Sacrum
Lateral

Patient Position
• Position patient lateral, with hips and knees flexed.

Part Position
• Support body to place long axis of spine horizontal.
• Prepare for positioning of central ray by centering sacrum to midline of grid.

Respiration:
Suspend.

Central Ray
• Perpendicular to level of ASIS and at a point 3½ inches (9 cm) posterior.
• Center IR to central ray.

Collimation:
Adjust to 10 × 12 inches (24 × 30 cm). Place side marker in the collimated exposure field.

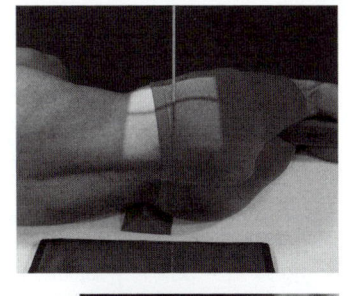

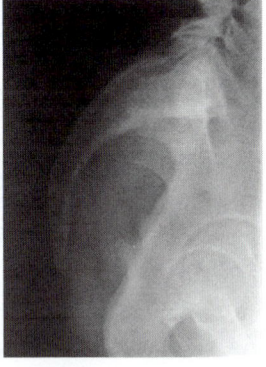

kVp: 96   *Reference: 14th edition ATLAS p. 1:487.*

Manual Factors

Part Thickness (cm)	mA	kVp	Time	mAs	SID	Image Receptor Size	CR, DR Exposure Indicator	Grid	HF, 1Ø or 3Ø

AEC Factors

Part Thickness (cm)	mA	kVp	AEC Detector	mAs	Density Comp.	Image Receptor Size	CR, DR Exposure Indicator	Grid	HF, 1Ø or 3Ø

Notes: _____ Competency: _____/____/____

Instructor: _____

Vertebral Column

Coccyx
AP axial

kVp: 85

Patient Position
- Position patient supine.

Part Position
- Center midsagittal plane to center of grid.

Respiration:
Suspend.

Central Ray
- Angle 10 degrees caudad and 2 inches (5 cm) superior to pubic symphysis.
- Center IR to central ray.

Collimation:
Adjust to 8 × 10 inches (18 × 24 cm). Place side marker in the collimated exposure field.

Reference: 14th edition ATLAS p. 1:486.

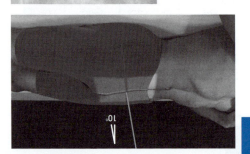

Manual Factors

Part Thickness (cm)	mA	kVp	Time	mAs	SID	Image Receptor Size	CR, DR Exposure Indicator	Grid	HF, 1Ø or 3Ø

AEC Factors

Part Thickness (cm)	mA	kVp	AEC Detector	mAs	Density Comp.	Image Receptor Size	CR, DR Exposure Indicator	Grid	HF, 1Ø or 3Ø

Notes: _____ Competency: ____/____/____

_____ Instructor: _____

Vertebral Column

Coccyx
Lateral

Patient Position
• Position patient lateral, with hips and knees flexed.

Part Position
• Support body to place long axis of spine horizontal.
• Prepare for positioning of central ray by centering coccyx to midline of grid.

Respiration:
Suspend.

Central Ray
• Perpendicular to a point 3½ inches (9 cm) posterior to ASIS and 2 inches (5 cm) inferior.
• Center IR to central ray.

Collimation:
Adjust to 6 × 8 inches (15 × 20 cm). Place side marker in the collimated exposure field.

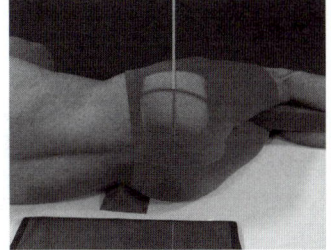

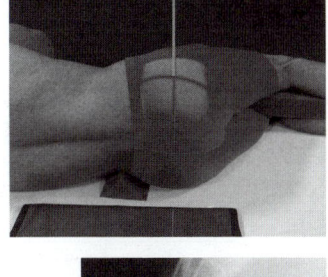

kVp: 85

Reference: 14th edition ATLAS p. 1:487.

Manual Factors

Part Thickness (cm)	mA	kVp	Time	mAs	SID	Image Receptor Size	CR, DR Exposure Indicator	Grid	HF, 1Ø or 3Ø

AEC Factors

Part Thickness (cm)	mA	kVp	AEC Detector	mAs	Density Comp.	Image Receptor Size	CR, DR Exposure Indicator	Grid	HF, 1Ø or 3Ø

Notes: _____ Competency: ____/____/____

Instructor: _____

Vertebral Column

Thoracolumbar Spine: Scoliosis
AP, PA, or lateral   FERGUSON METHOD

Patient Position
- Position patient upright, seated, or standing.

Part Position
- Position bottom of IR to include approximately 1 inch (2.5 cm) of iliac crests.
- Adjust midsagittal plane perpendicular to midline of grid.
- Have patient relax arms at sides.
- Obtain first image in normal upright position.
- Elevate foot or hip of convex side of curve 3 to 4 inches (8 to 10 cm) for second image.
- Do not support patient in this position.

Respiration
Suspend.

Central Ray
- Perpendicular to midpoint of IR.

Collimation:
Adjust to 12 × 17 inches (30 × 35 cm). Place side marker in the collimated exposure field.

kVp: 90

Reference: 14th edition ATLAS p. 1:495.

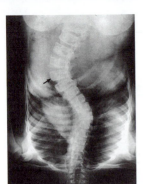

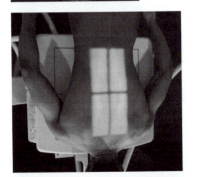

Manual Factors

Part Thickness (cm)	mA	kVp	Time	mAs	SID	Image Receptor Size	CR, DR Exposure Indicator	Grid	HF, 1Ø or 3Ø

AEC Factors

Part Thickness (cm)	mA	kVp	AEC Detector	mAs	Density Comp.	Image Receptor Size	CR, DR Exposure Indicator	Grid	HF, 1Ø or 3Ø

Notes: _____ Competency: ____/____/____

_____ Instructor: _____

Vertebral Column

Chest
PA, 186
Lateral, 188
PA oblique (LAO and RAO), 190
AP oblique (RPO and LPO), 192
AP, 194

Pulmonary Apices
AP axial (lordotic); LINDBLOM METHOD, 196

Lungs and Pleurae
AP or PA (lateral decubitus), 198
Lateral (dorsal or ventral decubitus), 200

Ribs
PA, 202
AP, 204
AP oblique (RPO or LPO), 206
PA oblique (RAO or LAO), 208

Sternum
PA oblique (RAO), 210
Lateral, 212

Thorax

Chest
PA

Patient Position
- Position patient standing or seated upright with back of hands on hips.

Part Position
- Center midsagittal plane with chin extended and eyes straight ahead.
- Have patient roll shoulders forward.
- Place top of IR 1½ to 2 inches (3.8 to 5 cm) above relaxed shoulders.
- Have patient flex arms and rest backs of hands on hips.
- Shield gonads.

Respiration:
Suspended full inspiration (after second inspiration).

Central Ray
- Perpendicular to the center of the IR. Use SID of 72 inches (183 cm).

Collimation:
Adjust to 14 × 17 inches (35 × 43 cm). Place side marker in the collimated exposure field.

kVp: 120

Reference: 14th edition ATLAS p. 1:107.

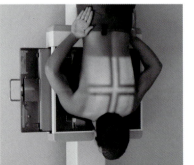
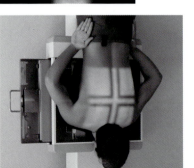

Manual Factors

Part Thickness (cm)	mA	kVp	Time	mAs	SID	Image Receptor Size	CR, DR Exposure Indicator	Grid	HF, 1Ø or 3Ø

AEC Factors

Part Thickness (cm)	mA	kVp	AEC Detector	mAs	Density Comp.	Image Receptor Size	CR, DR Exposure Indicator	Grid	HF, 1Ø or 3Ø

Notes: _____ Competency: ___/___/___

_____ Instructor: _____

Thorax

Chest
Lateral

Patient Position
• Position patient standing or seated upright with side against IR.

Part Position
• Place midsagittal plane parallel to IR.
• Have patient rest adjacent shoulder against IR holder, with arms raised and crossed over head.
• Place top of IR 1½ to 2 inches (3.8 to 5 cm) above shoulder.
• Center thorax to IR.
• Shield gonads.

Respiration:
Suspended full inspiration (after second inspiration).

Central Ray
• Direct perpendicular to IR, entering patient at level of T7. Use SID of 72 inches (183 cm).

Collimation:
Adjust to 14 × 17 inches (35 × 43 cm). Place side marker in the collimated exposure field.

kVp: 120

Reference: 14th edition ATLAS p. 1:110.

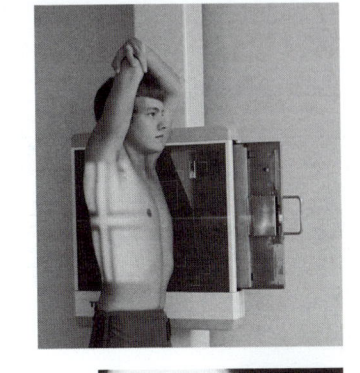

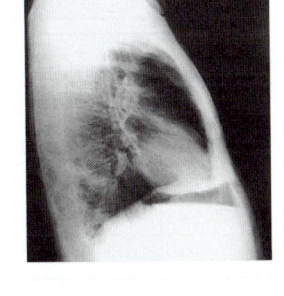

Manual Factors

Part Thickness (cm)	mA	kVp	Time	mAs	SID	Image Receptor Size	CR, DR Exposure Indicator	Grid	HF, 1Ø or 3Ø

AEC Factors

Part Thickness (cm)	mA	kVp	AEC Detector	mAs	Density Comp.	Image Receptor Size	CR, DR Exposure Indicator	Grid	HF, 1Ø or 3Ø

Notes: _____ Competency: ___/___/___

_____ Instructor: _____

Thorax

Chest
PA oblique (LAO and RAO)

Patient Position
• Position patient standing or seated upright. Side farther from IR is usually the side of primary interest.

Part Position
• Adjust coronal plane 45 degrees from plane of IR.
• Place top of IR 1½ to 2 inches (3.8 to 5 cm) above shoulders.
• Have patient roll shoulder nearest IR posteriorly and place hand on hip.
• Have patient place arm farther from IR on top of IR holder.
• Center thorax to IR. Both 45-degree obliques may be taken.
• Shield gonads.

Respiration:
Suspended full inspiration (after second inspiration).

Central Ray
• Perpendicular to IR at level of T7. Use SID of 72 inches (183 cm).

Collimation:
Adjust to 14 × 17 inches (35 × 43 cm). Place side marker in the collimated exposure field.

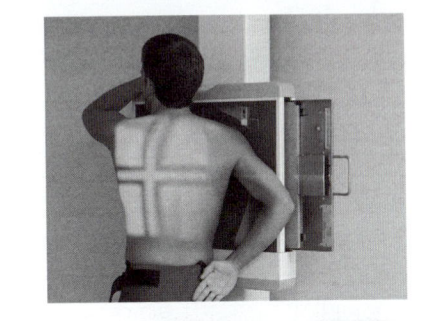

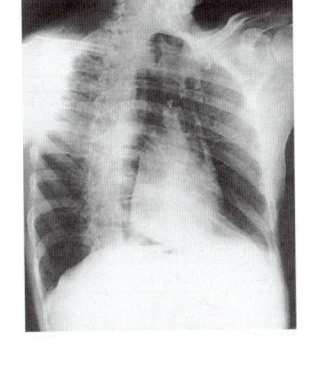

kVp: 120   *Reference: 14th edition ATLAS p. 1:113.*

Manual Factors

Part Thickness (cm)	mA	kVp	Time	mAs	SID	Image Receptor Size	CR, DR Exposure Indicator	Grid	HF, 1Ø or 3Ø

AEC Factors

Part Thickness (cm)	mA	kVp	AEC Detector	mAs	Density Comp.	Image Receptor Size	CR, DR Exposure Indicator	Grid	HF, 1Ø or 3Ø

Notes: _____ Competency: ____/____/____

_____ Instructor: _____

Thorax

Chest
AP oblique (RPO and LPO)

Patient Position
• Position patient upright or supine. Side closer to IR is usually side of primary interest.

Part Position
• Adjust coronal plane 45 degrees from plane of IR.
• Place top of IR 1½ to 2 inches (3.8 to 5 cm) above shoulders.
• Have patient roll shoulder nearest IR anteriorly and place hand on head.
• Have patient place arm farther from IR on hip.
• Center thorax to IR. Both 45-degree obliques may be taken.
• Shield gonads.

Respiration:
Suspended full inspiration (after second inspiration).

Central Ray
• Perpendicular to center of IR at a level 3 inches (8 cm) below jugular notch (level of T7). Use SID of 72 inches (183 cm), which is recommended measure.

Collimation:
Adjust to 14 × 17 inches (35 × 43 cm). Place side marker in the collimated exposure field.

kVp: 120

Reference: 14th edition ATLAS p. 1:117.

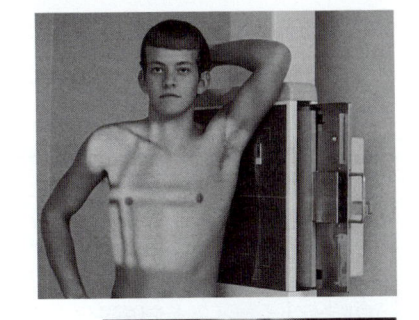

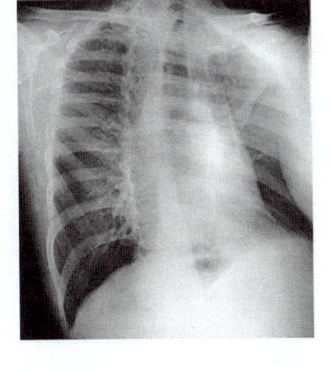

Manual Factors

Part Thickness (cm)	mA	kVp	Time	mAs	SID	Image Receptor Size	CR, DR Exposure Indicator	Grid	HF, 1Ø or 3Ø

AEC Factors

Part Thickness (cm)	mA	kVp	AEC Detector	mAs	Density Comp.	Image Receptor Size	CR, DR Exposure Indicator	Grid	HF, 1Ø or 3Ø

Notes: _____ Competency: _____/_____/_____

_____ Instructor: _____

Thorax

Chest
AP

Patient Position
• Position patient supine or upright, arms at sides.

Part Position
• Center IR to midsagittal plane, and adjust upper border to be 1½ to 2 inches (3.8 to 5 cm) above shoulders.
• If possible, have patient flex elbows, pronate hands, and place hands on hips.
• Shield gonads.

Respiration:
Suspended full inspiration (after second inspiration).

Central Ray
• Perpendicular to center of IR at level 3 inches (8 cm) below jugular notch (level of T7). Use SID of 72 inches (183 cm).

Collimation:
Adjust to 14 × 17 inches (35 × 43 cm). Place side marker in the collimated exposure field.

kVp: 90 (40" SID, non-grid), 105 (40", grid), 120 (72", grid) *Reference: 14th edition ATLAS p. 1:119.*

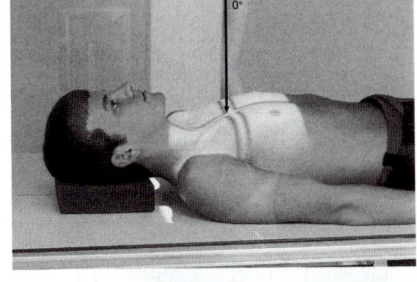

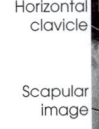

Manual Factors

Part Thickness (cm)	mA	kVp	Time	mAs	SID	Image Receptor Size	CR, DR Exposure Indicator	Grid	HF, 1Ø or 3Ø

AEC Factors

Part Thickness (cm)	mA	kVp	AEC Detector	mAs	Density Comp.	Image Receptor Size	CR, DR Exposure Indicator	Grid	HF, 1Ø or 3Ø

Notes: _____ Competency: ____/____/____

_____ Instructor: _____

Thorax

Pulmonary Apices
AP axial (lordotic)   LINDBLOM METHOD

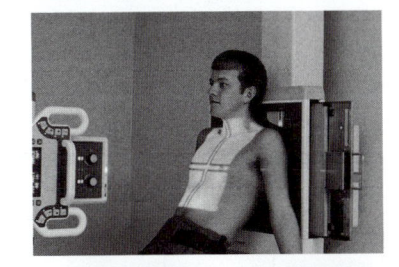

Patient Position
• Position patient standing, approximately 1 ft (30 cm) in front of IR. When patient is properly positioned, top of IR should be approximately 3 inches (8 cm) above shoulders.

Part Position
• Center midsagittal plane with no rotation.
• Have patient flex elbows, hands with palms out on hips.
• Have patient lean backward in extreme lordotic position.
• Shield gonads.

Respiration:
Suspended full inspiration (after second inspiration).

Central Ray
• Perpendicular to IR. Use SID of 72 inches (183 cm).

Collimation:
Adjust to 14 × 17 inches (35 × 43 cm). Place side marker in the collimated exposure field.

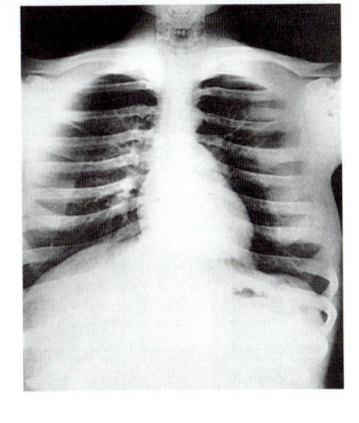

kVp: 120   *Reference: 14th edition ATLAS p. 1:121.*

Manual Factors

Part Thickness (cm)	mA	kVp	Time	mAs	SID	Image Receptor Size	CR, DR Exposure Indicator	Grid	HF, 1Ø or 3Ø

AEC Factors

Part Thickness (cm)	mA	kVp	AEC Detector	mAs	Density Comp.	Image Receptor Size	CR, DR Exposure Indicator	Grid	HF, 1Ø or 3Ø

Notes: _____ Competency: ____/____/____

_____ Instructor: _____

Thorax

Lungs and Pleurae
AP or PA (lateral decubitus)

Patient Position
• Position patient in lateral recumbent position.

Part Position
• Position patient on affected or unaffected side depending on condition.
• Elevate the chest on firm pad (typically "fluid down" or "free-air or pneumothorax up").
• Have patient extend arms above head; adjust thorax in true lateral position.
• Place top of IR approximately 1½ to 2 inches (3.8 to 5 cm) above shoulders.
• Shield gonads.

Respiration:
Suspended full inspiration (after second inspiration).

Central Ray
• Horizontal and perpendicular to center of IR at level 3 inches (8 cm) below jugular notch (at T7 for PA).

Collimation:
Adjust to 14 × 17 inches (35 × 43 cm). Place side marker in the collimated exposure field.

kVp: 120

Reference: 14th edition ATLAS p. 1:125.

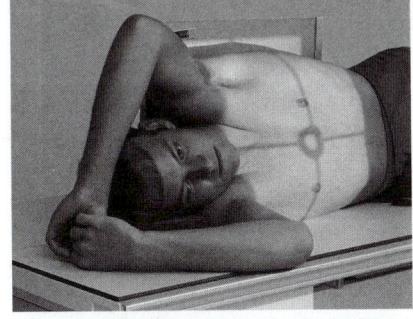

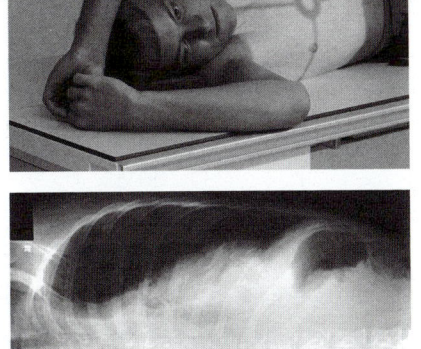

Manual Factors

Part Thickness (cm)	mA	kVp	Time	mAs	SID	Image Receptor Size	CR, DR Exposure Indicator	Grid	HF, 1Ø or 3Ø

AEC Factors

Part Thickness (cm)	mA	kVp	AEC Detector	mAs	Density Comp.	Image Receptor Size	CR, DR Exposure Indicator	Grid	HF, 1Ø or 3Ø

Notes: _____ Competency: _____/_____/_____

Instructor: _____

Thorax

Lungs and Pleurae
Lateral (dorsal or ventral decubitus)

Patient Position
• Position patient prone or supine.

Part Position
• Elevate thorax 2 to 3 inches (5 to 8 cm) on firm pad, and center with affected side closer to IR.
• Have patient extend arms above head.
• Place top of IR 1½ to 2 inches (3.8 to 5 cm) above top of shoulders.
• Center midcoronal plane to center of grid.
• Shield gonads.

Respiration:
Suspended full inspiration (after second inspiration).

Central Ray
• Horizontal and centered to IR at level of midcoronal plane and 3 inches (8 cm) below jugular notch (T7 for ventral decubitus)

Collimation:
Adjust to 14 × 17 inches (35 × 43 cm). Place side marker in the collimated exposure field.

kVp: 120

Reference: 14th edition ATLAS p. 1:127.

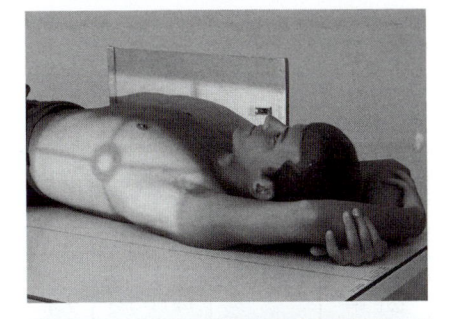

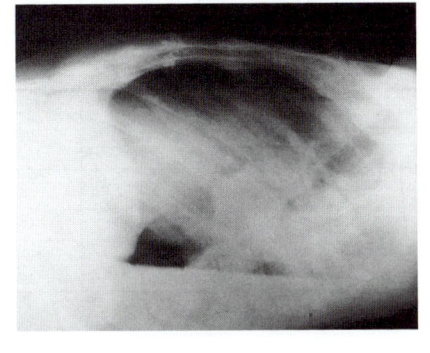

Manual Factors

Part Thickness (cm)	mA	kVp	Time	mAs	SID	Image Receptor Size	CR, DR Exposure Indicator	Grid	HF, 1Ø or 3Ø

AEC Factors

Part Thickness (cm)	mA	kVp	AEC Detector	mAs	Density Comp.	Image Receptor Size	CR, DR Exposure Indicator	Grid	HF, 1Ø or 3Ø

Notes: _____ Competency: _____/_____/_____

_____ Instructor: _____

Thorax

Ribs
PA

Patient Position
• Position patient upright or prone.

Part Position
• Center midsagittal plane to grid with chin extended and eyes straight ahead.
• Place top of IR approximately 1½ inches (3.8 cm) above shoulders.
• Have patient roll shoulders forward and rest back of hands on hips.
• Shield gonads.

Respiration:
Suspended full inspiration to depress diaphragm.

Central Ray
• Perpendicular to center of IR. This places the central ray at level of T7.

Collimation:
Adjust to 14 × 17 inches (35 × 43 cm). Place side marker in the collimated exposure field.

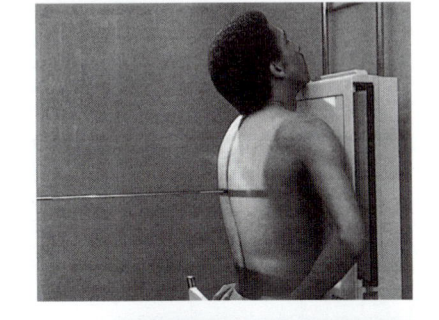

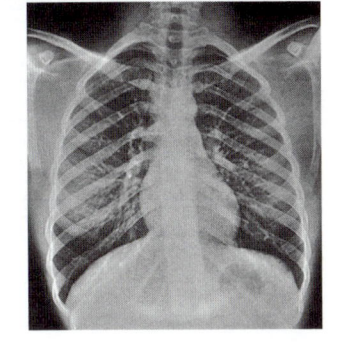

kVp: 80

Reference: 14th edition ATLAS p. 1:527.

Manual Factors

Part Thickness (cm)	mA	kVp	Time	mAs	SID	Image Receptor Size	CR, DR Exposure Indicator	Grid	HF, 1Ø or 3Ø

AEC Factors

Part Thickness (cm)	mA	kVp	AEC Detector	mAs	Density Comp.	Image Receptor Size	CR, DR Exposure Indicator	Grid	HF, 1Ø or 3Ø

Notes: _____ Competency: ____/____/____

_____ Instructor: _____

Thorax

Ribs
AP

Patient Position
• Position patient upright or supine.

Part Position
• Center midsagittal plane to midline of grid.
• *Above diaphragm*: Place top of IR 1½ inches (3.8 cm) above relaxed shoulders.
• *Below diaphragm*: Center thorax with bottom of IR near level of iliac crests.
• Rotate shoulders anteriorly.
• Shield gonads.

Respiration:
Above diaphragm: Suspended full inspiration.
Below diaphragm: Suspended full expiration.

Central Ray
• Perpendicular to center of IR.

Collimation:
Adjust to 14 × 17 inches (35 × 43 cm). Place side marker in the collimated exposure field.

kVp: 80   *Reference: 14th edition ATLAS p. 1:529.*

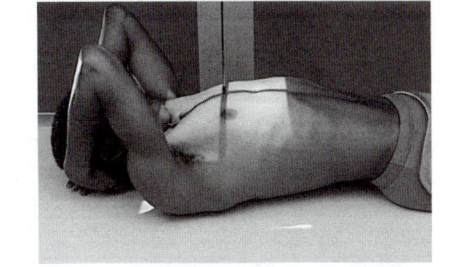

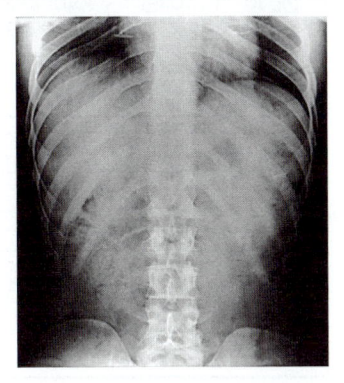

Manual Factors

Part Thickness (cm)	mA	kVp	Time	mAs	SID	Image Receptor Size	CR, DR Exposure Indicator	Grid	HF, 1Ø or 3Ø

AEC Factors

Part Thickness (cm)	mA	kVp	AEC Detector	mAs	Density Comp.	Image Receptor Size	CR, DR Exposure Indicator	Grid	HF, 1Ø or 3Ø

Notes: _____

Competency: ____/____/____

Instructor: _____

Thorax

Ribs
AP oblique (RPO or LPO)

Patient Position
• Position patient upright or supine.

Part Position
• Rotate patient's body 45 degrees with affected side toward IR.
• Center a plane midway between midsagittal plane and lateral surface of body.
• Position arms clear of thorax. Center top of IR 1½ inches (3.8 cm) above relaxed shoulder (for above diaphragm) and with lower edge of IR near level of iliac crest (for below diaphragm).
• Shield gonads.

Respiration:
Above diaphragm: Suspended full inspiration.
Below diaphragm: Suspended full expiration.

Central Ray
• Perpendicular to center of IR.

Collimation:
Adjust to 14 × 17 inches (35 × 43 cm). Place side marker in the collimated exposure field.

kVp: 80   *Reference: 14th edition ATLAS p. 1:531.*

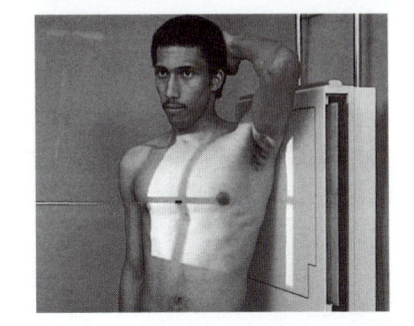

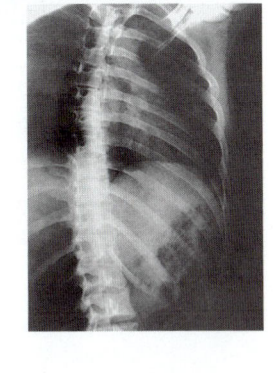

Manual Factors

Part Thickness (cm)	mA	kVp	Time	mAs	SID	Image Receptor Size	CR, DR Exposure Indicator	Grid	HF, 1Ø or 3Ø

AEC Factors

Part Thickness (cm)	mA	kVp	AEC Detector	mAs	Density Comp.	Image Receptor Size	CR, DR Exposure Indicator	Grid	HF, 1Ø or 3Ø

Notes: _____ Competency: _____/____/____

_____ Instructor: _____

Thorax

Ribs
PA oblique (RAO or LAO)

Patient Position
• Position patient upright or prone.

Part Position
• Rotate patient's body 45 degrees with affected side away from IR.
• Center a plane midway between midsagittal plane and lateral body surface.
• Position arms clear of thorax. Center top of IR 1½ inches (3.8 cm) above relaxed shoulder (for above diaphragm) and with lower edge of IR near level of iliac crest (for below diaphragm).
• Shield gonads.

Respiration:
Above diaphragm: Suspended full inspiration.
Below diaphragm: Suspended full expiration.

Central Ray
• Perpendicular to center of IR.

Collimation:
Adjust to 14 × 17 inches (35 × 43 cm). Place side marker in the collimated exposure field.

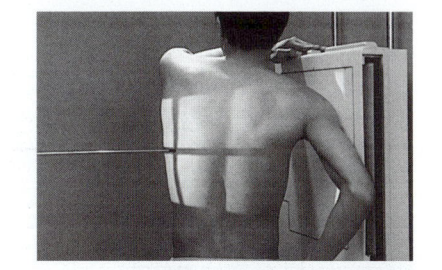

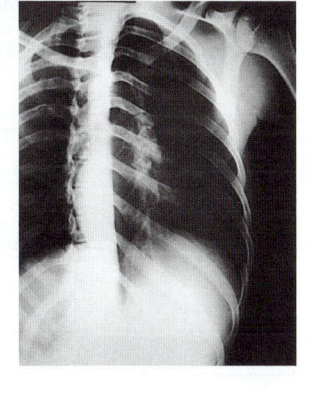

kVp: 80   *Reference: 14th edition ATLAS p. 1:533.*

Manual Factors

Part Thickness (cm)	mA	kVp	Time	mAs	SID	Image Receptor Size	CR, DR Exposure Indicator	Grid	HF, 1Ø or 3Ø

AEC Factors

Part Thickness (cm)	mA	kVp	AEC Detector	mAs	Density Comp.	Image Receptor Size	CR, DR Exposure Indicator	Grid	HF, 1Ø or 3Ø

Notes: _____ Competency: _____/____/____

Instructor: _____

Thorax

Sternum
PA oblique (RAO)

Patient Position
• Position patient prone for RAO (right PA oblique).

Part Position
• Center sternum to grid.
• Rotate patient's body 15 to 20 degrees to prevent superimposition of vertebral and sternal images.
• Center IR midway between jugular notch and xiphoid process at level of T7.
• Shield gonads.

Respiration:
Shallow breathing or suspended expiration.

Central Ray
• Perpendicular to T7. Central ray enters elevated side of posterior thorax approximately 1 inch (2.5 cm) lateral to midsagittal plane.

Collimation:
Adjust to 10 × 12 inches (24 × 30 cm). Place side marker in the collimated exposure field.

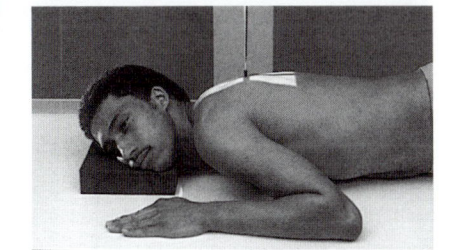

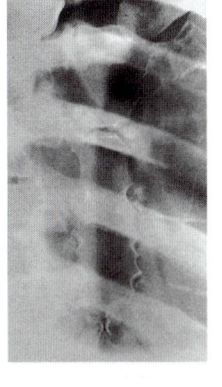

kVp: 80   *Reference: 14th edition ATLAS p. 1:516.*

Manual Factors

Part Thickness (cm)	mA	kVp	Time	mAs	SID	Image Receptor Size	CR, DR Exposure Indicator	Grid	HF, 1Ø or 3Ø

AEC Factors

Part Thickness (cm)	mA	kVp	AEC Detector	mAs	Density Comp.	Image Receptor Size	CR, DR Exposure Indicator	Grid	HF, 1Ø or 3Ø

Notes: _____ Competency: _____/____/____

_____ Instructor: _____

Thorax

Sternum
Lateral

Patient Position
• Position patient seated, standing lateral, or recumbent.

Part Position
• Place top of IR 1½ inches (3.8 cm) above jugular notch.
• Have patient rotate shoulders and arms posteriorly for upright positioning; place arms above head for recumbent positioning.
• Center sternum to grid. Adjust to true lateral position.
• Shield gonads.

Respiration:
Suspended deep inspiration.

Central Ray
• Perpendicular to center of IR, entering lateral border of midsternum. Use SID of 72 inches (183 cm).

Collimation:
Adjust to 10 × 12 inches (24 × 30 cm). Place side marker in the collimated exposure field.

kVp: 80   *Reference: 14th edition ATLAS p. 1:520.*

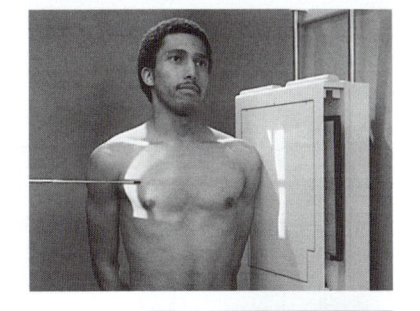

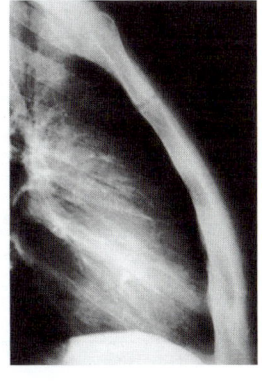

Manual Factors

Part Thickness (cm)	mA	kVp	Time	mAs	SID	Image Receptor Size	CR, DR Exposure Indicator	Grid	HF, 1Ø or 3Ø

AEC Factors

Part Thickness (cm)	mA	kVp	AEC Detector	mAs	Density Comp.	Image Receptor Size	CR, DR Exposure Indicator	Grid	HF, 1Ø or 3Ø

Notes: _____ Competency: ____/____/____

Instructor: _____

Thorax

Abdomen:
- AP (supine), 216
- AP (upright), 218
- AP (lateral decubitus), 220
- Lateral, 222
- Lateral (dorsal decubitus), 224

Esophagus:
- AP or PA, 226
- PA oblique (RAO), 228
- Lateral, 230

Stomach and Duodenum:
- PA, 232
- PA oblique (RAO), 234
- AP oblique (LPO), 236
- Lateral, 238
- AP, 240

Small Intestine:
- AP or PA, 242

Large Intestine:
- PA, 244
- PA axial, 246
- PA oblique (LAO and RAO), 248
- Lateral, 250
- AP, 252
- AP axial, 254
- AP oblique (LPO and RPO), 256
- AP or PA (lateral decubitus), 258
- Lateral, AP or PA, oblique (upright), 260

Urinary System:
- AP oblique (RPO and LPO), 262

Bladder:
- AP or PA axial, 264
- AP oblique (RPO or LPO), 266
- Lateral, 268

Abdomen

Abdomen
AP (supine)

Patient Position
- Position patient supine.

Part Position
- Center midsagittal plane to grid.
- Maintain shoulders in same transverse plane.
- Support under knees.
- Center IR at level of iliac crests, and ensure that pubic symphysis is included.
- Apply gonad shielding as appropriate.

Respiration:
Suspend.

Central Ray
- Perpendicular to IR midline at level of iliac crests.

Collimation:
Adjust to 14 × 17 inches (35 × 43 cm). Place side marker in the collimated exposure field.

kVp: 85

Reference: 14th edition ATLAS p. 1:137.

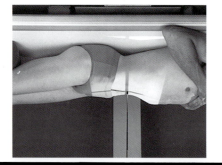
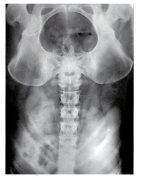

Manual Factors

Part Thickness (cm)	mA	kVp	Time	mAs	SID	Image Receptor Size	CR, DR Exposure Indicator	Grid	HF, 1Ø or 3Ø

AEC Factors

Part Thickness (cm)	mA	kVp	AEC Detector	mAs	Density Comp.	Image Receptor Size	CR, DR Exposure Indicator	Grid	HF, 1Ø or 3Ø

Notes: _____ Competency: _____/_____/_____

_____ Instructor: _____

Abdomen

Abdomen
AP (upright)

Patient Position
• Position patient upright.

Part Position
• Center midsagittal plane to grid device.
• Maintain shoulders in same transverse plane.
• Center IR 2 inches (5 cm) above iliac crests to include diaphragm.
• Apply gonad shielding as appropriate.

Respiration:
Suspend.

Central Ray
• Horizontal and 2 inches (5 cm) superior to iliac crests to center of IR.

Collimation:
Adjust to 14 × 17 inches (35 × 43 cm). Place side marker in the collimated exposure field.

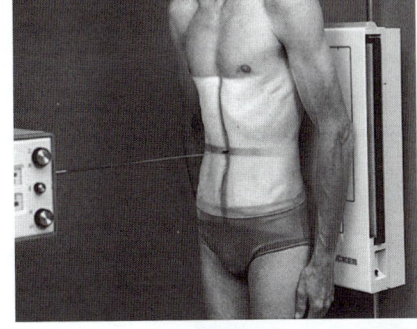

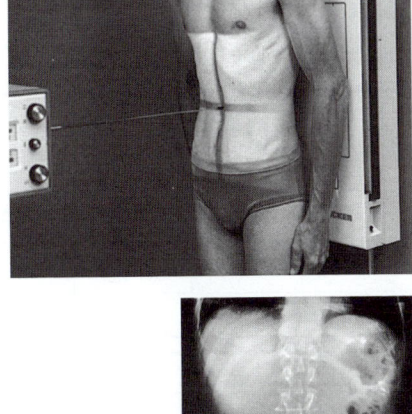

kVp: 85

Reference: 14th edition ATLAS p. 1:137.

Manual Factors

Part Thickness (cm)	mA	kVp	Time	mAs	SID	Image Receptor Size	CR, DR Exposure Indicator	Grid	HF, 1Ø or 3Ø

AEC Factors

Part Thickness (cm)	mA	kVp	AEC Detector	mAs	Density Comp.	Image Receptor Size	CR, DR Exposure Indicator	Grid	HF, 1Ø or 3Ø

Notes: _____ Competency: _____/_____/_____

_____ Instructor: _____

Abdomen

Abdomen
AP (lateral decubitus)

Patient Position
- Position patient in lateral recumbent position (usually left side down) on pad.
- Place patient's arms above level of diaphragm, with knees slightly flexed.

Part Position
- Adjust midsagittal plane perpendicular to and centered to grid device.
- Center IR at level of iliac crests.
- Center 2 inches (5 cm) above iliac crests if diaphragm is to be included.
- Apply gonad shielding as appropriate.

Respiration:
Suspend.

Central Ray
- Horizontal and perpendicular to midpoint of IR.
NOTE: Show side up for air and side down for fluid.

Collimation:
Adjust to 14 × 17 inches (35 × 43 cm). Place side marker in the collimated exposure field.

kVp: 85   *Reference: 14th edition ATLAS p. 1:139.*

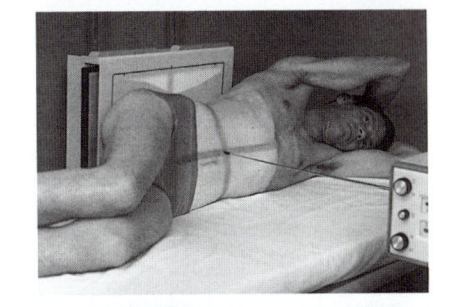

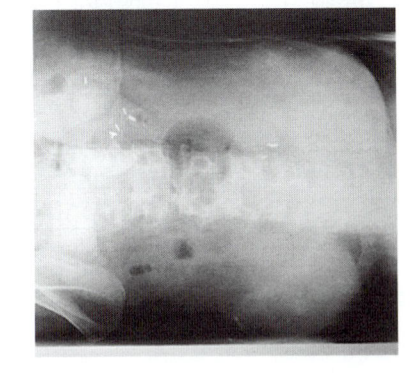

Manual Factors

Part Thickness (cm)	mA	kVp	Time	mAs	SID	Image Receptor Size	CR, DR Exposure Indicator	Grid	HF, 1Ø or 3Ø

AEC Factors

Part Thickness (cm)	mA	kVp	AEC Detector	mAs	Density Comp.	Image Receptor Size	CR, DR Exposure Indicator	Grid	HF, 1Ø or 3Ø

Notes: _____ Competency: ____/____/____

Instructor: _____

Abdomen

Abdomen
Lateral

Patient Position
• Position patient in lateral recumbent position or upright.

Part Position
• Center midcoronal plane to grid.
• Have patient flex elbows and place hands under head.
• Center IR at level of iliac crests or approximately 2 inches (5 cm) superior to crests if diaphragm is to be included.
• Shield gonads.

Respiration:
Suspend.

Central Ray
• Perpendicular to midpoint of IR.

Collimation:
Adjust to 14 × 17 inches (35 × 43 cm). Place side marker in the collimated exposure field.

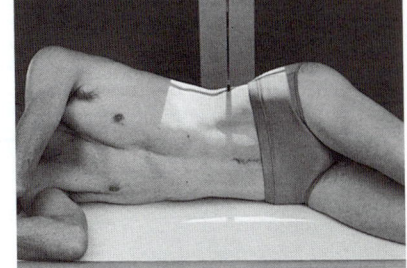

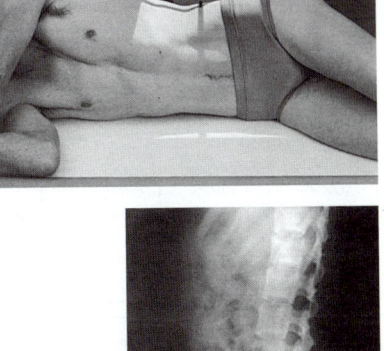

kVp: 90

Reference: 14th edition ATLAS p. 1:141.

Manual Factors

Part Thickness (cm)	mA	kVp	Time	mAs	SID	Image Receptor Size	CR, DR Exposure Indicator	Grid	HF, 1Ø or 3Ø

AEC Factors

Part Thickness (cm)	mA	kVp	AEC Detector	mAs	Density Comp.	Image Receptor Size	CR, DR Exposure Indicator	Grid	HF, 1Ø or 3Ø

Notes: _____

Competency: ____/____/____

Instructor: _____

Abdomen

Abdomen
Lateral (dorsal decubitus)

Patient Position
• Position patient supine.

Part Position
• Have patient place arms across upper chest or under head. Patient may slightly flex knees.
• Center vertical grid device to midcoronal plane at level 2 inches (5 cm) superior to iliac crests.
• Shield gonads.

Respiration:
Suspend.

Central Ray
• Horizontal and perpendicular to center of IR, entering midcoronal plane 2 inches (5 cm) above iliac crests.

Collimation:
Adjust to 14 × 17 inches (35 × 43 cm). Place side marker in the collimated exposure field.

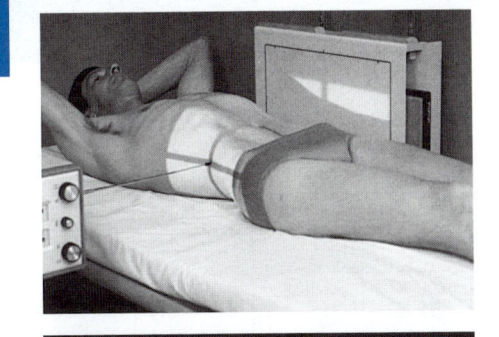

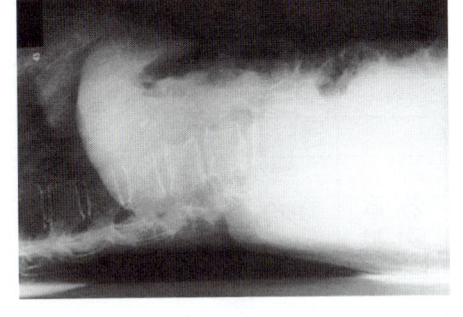

kVp: 90

Reference: 14th edition ATLAS p. 1:142.

Manual Factors

Part Thickness (cm)	mA	kVp	Time	mAs	SID	Image Receptor Size	CR, DR Exposure Indicator	Grid	HF, 1Ø or 3Ø

AEC Factors

Part Thickness (cm)	mA	kVp	AEC Detector	mAs	Density Comp.	Image Receptor Size	CR, DR Exposure Indicator	Grid	HF, 1Ø or 3Ø

Notes: _____ Competency: ____/____/____

_____ Instructor: _____

Abdomen

Esophagus
AP or PA

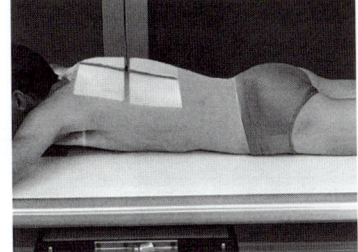

Patient Position
• Position patient supine or prone.

Part Position
• Center midsagittal plane to grid.
• Have patient place arms above the head in a comfortable position.
• Adjust shoulders and hips equidistant from table.
• Place top of IR at level of mouth.
• Turn head slightly to facilitate drinking barium mixture, and give barium to patient.

Respiration:
Suspend.

Central Ray
• Perpendicular to midpoint of IR at level of T5-T6.

Collimation:
Adjust to 12 × 17 inches (30 × 43 cm). Place side marker in the collimated exposure field.

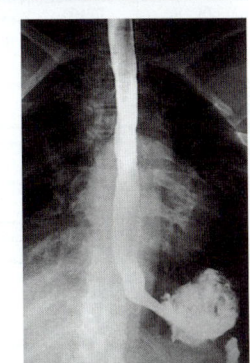

kVp: 120

Reference: 14th edition ATLAS p. 2:218.

Manual Factors

Part Thickness (cm)	mA	kVp	Time	mAs	SID	Image Receptor Size	CR, DR Exposure Indicator	Grid	HF, 1Ø or 3Ø

AEC Factors

Part Thickness (cm)	mA	kVp	AEC Detector	mAs	Density Comp.	Image Receptor Size	CR, DR Exposure Indicator	Grid	HF, 1Ø or 3Ø

Notes: _____ Competency: ____/____/____

Instructor: _____

Abdomen

Esophagus
PA oblique (RAO)

Patient Position
• Position patient recumbent with the side-down arm at the side and the side-up arm on the pillow.

Part Position
• Elevate left side to obliquity of 35 to 40 degrees.
• Support patient on flexed knee and elbow.
• Place top of IR at level of mouth.
• Align esophagus and center elevated side through plane 2 inches (5 cm) lateral to midsagittal plane; give barium to patient.
• Shield gonads.

Respiration:
Suspend.

Central Ray
• Perpendicular to midpoint of IR at level of T5 or T6.
NOTE: If patient cannot assume prone position, a similar image can be obtained by using LPO position, modified as described previously.

Collimation:
Adjust to 12 × 17 inches (30 × 43 cm). Place side marker in the collimated exposure field.

kVp: 120

Reference: 14th edition ATLAS p. 2-218

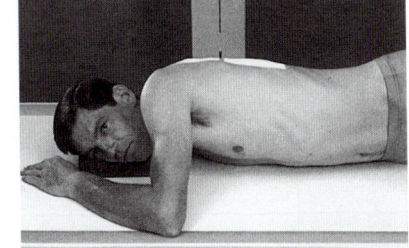

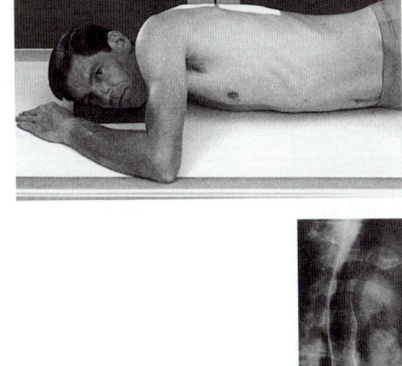

Manual Factors									
Part Thickness (cm)	mA	kVp	Time	mAs	SID	Image Receptor Size	CR, DR Exposure Indicator	Grid	HF, 1Ø or 3Ø

AEC Factors									
Part Thickness (cm)	mA	kVp	AEC Detector	mAs	Density Comp.	Image Receptor Size	CR, DR Exposure Indicator	Grid	HF, 1Ø or 3Ø

Notes: _____ Competency: ____/____/____

Instructor: _____

Abdomen

Esophagus
Lateral

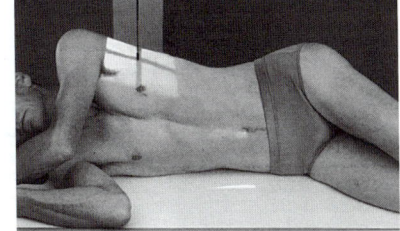

Patient Position
• Place patient's arms forward, with forearm on the pillow near the head.

Part Position
• Center midcoronal plane to grid.
• Have patient bring arms forward and slightly flex hips and knees.
• Place top of film at level of mouth.
• Give barium mixture to patient.
• Shield gonads.

Respiration:
Suspend.

Central Ray
• Perpendicular to midpoint of IR at level of T5-T6.

Collimation:
Adjust to 12 × 17 inches (30 × 43 cm). Place side marker in the collimated exposure field.

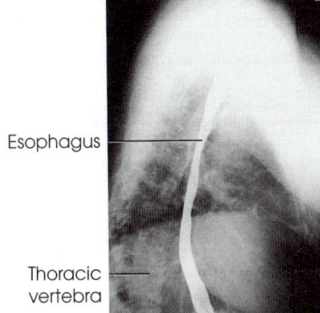

kVp: 120   *Reference: 14th edition ATLAS p. 2:218.*

Manual Factors									
Part Thickness (cm)	mA	kVp	Time	mAs	SID	Image Receptor Size	CR, DR Exposure Indicator	Grid	HF, 1Ø or 3Ø

AEC Factors									
Part Thickness (cm)	mA	kVp	AEC Detector	mAs	Density Comp.	Image Receptor Size	CR, DR Exposure Indicator	Grid	HF, 1Ø or 3Ø

Notes: _____ Competency: ____/____/____

Instructor: _____

Abdomen

Stomach and Duodenum
PA

Patient Position
• Position patient prone.

Part Position
• Center IR at estimated level of L1-L2.
• Center (1) halfway between midline and left lateral border of abdominal cavity for 10- × 12-inch (24- × 30-cm) IR or (2) in midsagittal plane for 14- × 17-inch (35- × 43-cm) IR.
• Shield gonads.

Respiration:
Suspend.

Central Ray
• Perpendicular to IR at level of L1-L2.

Collimation:
Adjust to 10 × 12 inches (24 × 30 cm) or 11 × 14 inches (28 × 36 cm). Place side marker in the collimated exposure field.

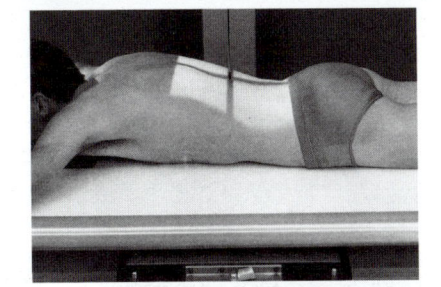

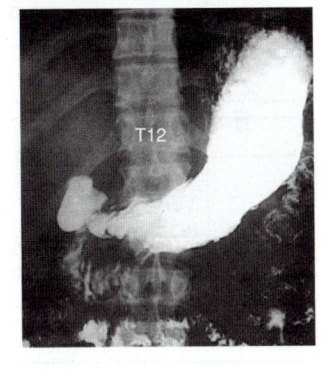

kVp: 120　　　　　　*Reference: 14th edition ATLAS p. 2:223.*

Manual Factors

Part Thickness (cm)	mA	kVp	Time	mAs	SID	Image Receptor Size	CR, DR Exposure Indicator	Grid	HF, 1Ø or 3Ø

AEC Factors

Part Thickness (cm)	mA	kVp	AEC Detector	mAs	Density Comp.	Image Receptor Size	CR, DR Exposure Indicator	Grid	HF, 1Ø or 3Ø

Notes: _____ Competency: ____/____/____

Instructor: _____

Abdomen

Stomach and Duodenum
PA oblique (RAO)

Patient Position
- Position patient recumbent with the right arm at the side and left arm by the head.

Part Position
- Elevate left side, and support patient to obliquity of 40 to 70 degrees. (Hypersthenic patients require the greatest rotation.)
- Center IR at level of L1-L2.
- Position patient so that a sagittal plane passing midway between vertebrae and lateral border of elevated side is centered to grid.
- Shield gonads.

Respiration:
Suspend.

Central Ray
- Perpendicular to center of IR midway between vertebral column and lateral border of abdomen at level of L1-L2.

Collimation:
Adjust to 10 × 12 inches (24 × 30 cm) or 11 × 14 inches (28 × 36 cm). Place side marker in the collimated exposure field.

kVp: 120

Reference: 14th edition ATLAS p. 2:226.

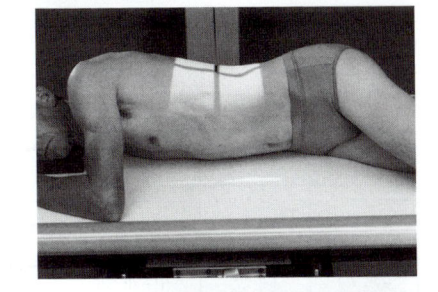

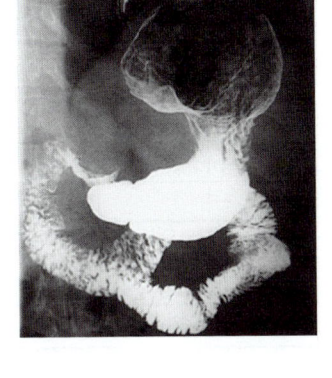

Manual Factors

Part Thickness (cm)	mA	kVp	Time	mAs	SID	Image Receptor Size	CR, DR Exposure Indicator	Grid	HF, 1Ø or 3Ø

AEC Factors

Part Thickness (cm)	mA	kVp	AEC Detector	mAs	Density Comp.	Image Receptor Size	CR, DR Exposure Indicator	Grid	HF, 1Ø or 3Ø

Notes: _____ Competency: ____/____/____

_____ Instructor: _____

Abdomen

Stomach and Duodenum
AP oblique (LPO)

Patient Position
• Position patient recumbent with left arm by head and right arm behind body.

Part Position
• Elevate right side, and support patient to obliquity of 30 to 60 degrees. (Hypersthenic patients require the greatest rotation; 45 degrees is sufficient for asthenic patients.)
• Position patient so that sagittal plane passing midway between vertebrae and left margin of abdomen is centered to IR.
• Center IR at level of L1-L2.
• Shield gonads.

Respiration:
Suspend.

Central Ray
• Perpendicular to center of IR midway between vertebral column and left lateral border of abdomen at level of L1-L2.

Collimation:
Adjust to 10 × 12 inches (24 × 30 cm) or 11 × 14 inches (28 × 36 cm). Place side marker in the collimated exposure field.

kVp: 120   Reference: 14th edition ATLAS p. 2:228

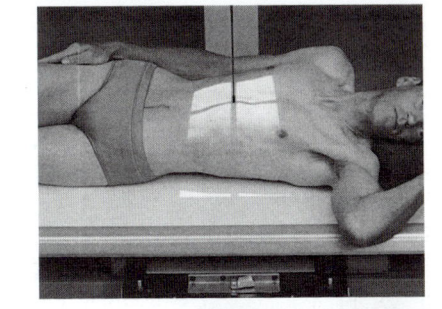

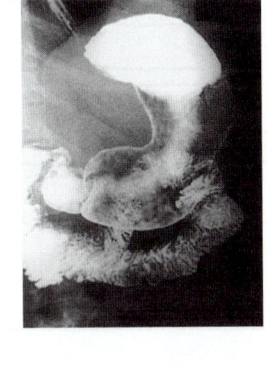

Manual Factors

Part Thickness (cm)	mA	kVp	Time	mAs	SID	Image Receptor Size	CR, DR Exposure Indicator	Grid	HF, 1Ø or 3Ø

AEC Factors

Part Thickness (cm)	mA	kVp	AEC Detector	mAs	Density Comp.	Image Receptor Size	CR, DR Exposure Indicator	Grid	HF, 1Ø or 3Ø

Notes: _____ Competency: _____/_____/_____

Instructor: _____

Abdomen

Stomach and Duodenum
Lateral

Patient Position
• Position patient recumbent (right lateral) or upright (left lateral).

Part Position
• Adjust body so that plane passing between midcoronal plane and anterior abdominal surface is centered to grid.
• Center IR at level of L1-L2.
• Adjust to true lateral.
• Shield gonads.

Respiration:
Suspend.

Central Ray
• Perpendicular to center of IR midway between midcoronal plane and anterior surface of abdomen at level of L1-L2 for recumbent or L3 for upright position.

Collimation:
Adjust to 10 × 12 inches (24 × 30 cm) or 11 × 14 inches (28 × 36 cm). Place side marker in the collimated exposure field.

kVp: 120

Reference: 14th edition ATLAS p. 2:230.

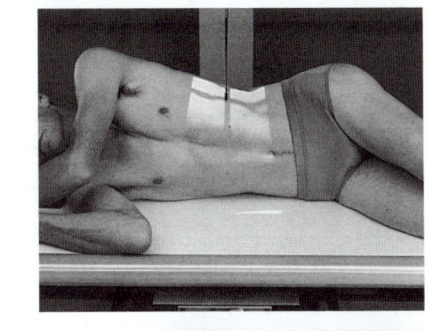

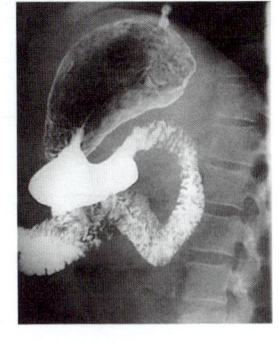

Manual Factors

Part Thickness (cm)	mA	kVp	Time	mAs	SID	Image Receptor Size	CR, DR Exposure Indicator	Grid	HF, 1Ø or 3Ø

AEC Factors

Part Thickness (cm)	mA	kVp	AEC Detector	mAs	Density Comp.	Image Receptor Size	CR, DR Exposure Indicator	Grid	HF, 1Ø or 3Ø

Notes: _____ Competency: _____/___/___

Instructor: _____

Abdomen

Stomach and Duodenum
AP

Patient Position
• Position patient supine.

Part Position
• Adjust patient so that midline of grid coincides (1) halfway between midline and lateral border of abdomen for 10- × 12-inch (24- × 30-cm) IR or (2) at midsagittal plane for 14- × 17-inch (35- × 43-cm) IR.
• Center IR at level of L1-L2.
• Shield gonads.

Respiration:
Suspend.

Central Ray
• Perpendicular to IR at level of pylorus (L1-L2).

Collimation:
Adjust to 10 × 12 inches (24 × 30 cm) or 14 × 17 inches (35 × 43 cm). Place side marker in the collimated exposure field.

kVp: 120   *Reference: 14th edition ATLAS p. 2:232.*

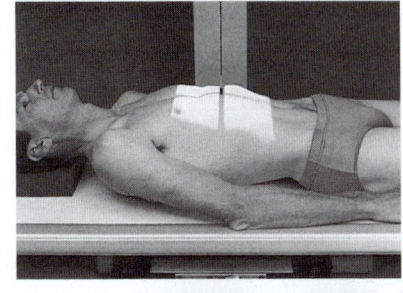

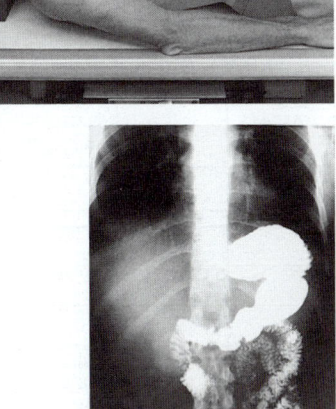

Manual Factors

Part Thickness (cm)	mA	kVp	Time	mAs	SID	Image Receptor Size	CR, DR Exposure Indicator	Grid	HF, 1Ø or 3Ø

AEC Factors

Part Thickness (cm)	mA	kVp	AEC Detector	mAs	Density Comp.	Image Receptor Size	CR, DR Exposure Indicator	Grid	HF, 1Ø or 3Ø

Notes: _____ Competency: _____/_____/_____

_____ Instructor: _____

Abdomen

Small Intestine
AP or PA

Patient Position
• Position patient supine or prone.

Part Position
• Center midsagittal plane to grid.
• Center IR at level of iliac crests (may be slightly higher for early time exposures).
• Shield gonads.

Respiration:
Suspend.

Central Ray
• Perpendicular to IR, entering level of iliac crests (or slightly above).

Collimation:
Adjust to 14 × 17 inches (35 × 43 cm). Place side marker in the collimated exposure field.

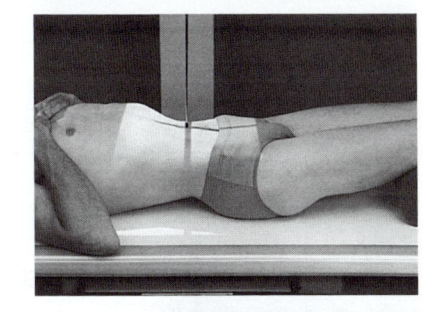

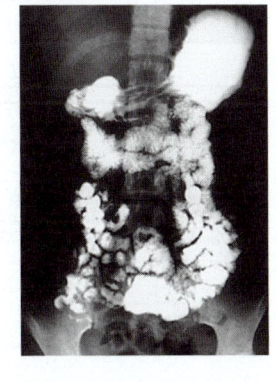

kVp: 120

Reference: 14th edition ATLAS p. 2:237.

Manual Factors

Part Thickness (cm)	mA	kVp	Time	mAs	SID	Image Receptor Size	CR, DR Exposure Indicator	Grid	HF, 1Ø or 3Ø

AEC Factors

Part Thickness (cm)	mA	kVp	AEC Detector	mAs	Density Comp.	Image Receptor Size	CR, DR Exposure Indicator	Grid	HF, 1Ø or 3Ø

Notes: _____ Competency: _____/_____/_____

_____ Instructor: _____

Abdomen

Large Intestine
PA

Patient Position
• Position patient prone.

Part Position
• Center midsagittal plane to grid.
• Center IR at level of iliac crests.
• Shield gonads.

Respiration:
Suspend.

Central Ray
• Perpendicular to IR, entering level of iliac crests.

Collimation:
Adjust to 14 × 17 inches (35 × 43 cm). Place side marker in the collimated exposure field.

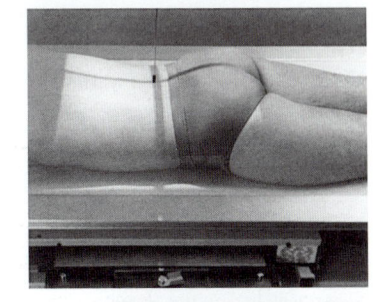

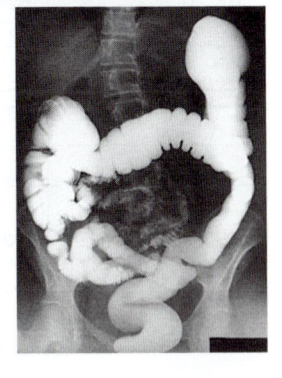

kVp: 120   *Reference: 14th edition ATLAS p. 2:250.*

Manual Factors

Part Thickness (cm)	mA	kVp	Time	mAs	SID	Image Receptor Size	CR, DR Exposure Indicator	Grid	HF, 1Ø or 3Ø

AEC Factors

Part Thickness (cm)	mA	kVp	AEC Detector	mAs	Density Comp.	Image Receptor Size	CR, DR Exposure Indicator	Grid	HF, 1Ø or 3Ø

Notes: _____ Competency: ____/____/____

Instructor: _____

Abdomen

Large Intestine
PA axial

Patient Position
• Position patient prone.

Part Position
• Center midsagittal plane to grid with center of IR at level of iliac crests.
• Shield gonads.

Respiration:
Suspend.

Central Ray
• Angle 30 to 40 degrees caudad. To show retrosigmoid area using smaller IR, direct central ray so that it enters midline at level of ASIS.

Collimation:
Adjust to 14 × 17 inches (35 × 43 cm). Place side marker in the collimated exposure field.

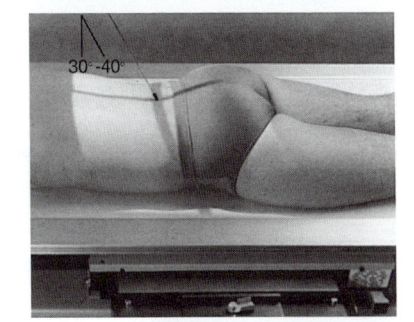

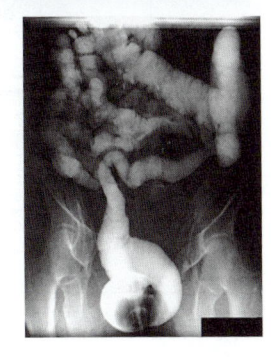

kVp: 120

Reference: 14th edition ATLAS p. 2:252.

Manual Factors

Part Thickness (cm)	mA	kVp	Time	mAs	SID	Image Receptor Size	CR, DR Exposure Indicator	Grid	HF, 1Ø or 3Ø

AEC Factors

Part Thickness (cm)	mA	kVp	AEC Detector	mAs	Density Comp.	Image Receptor Size	CR, DR Exposure Indicator	Grid	HF, 1Ø or 3Ø

Notes: _____ Competency: _____/___/___

_____ Instructor: _____

Abdomen

Large Intestine
PA oblique (LAO and RAO)

Patient Position
• Position patient PA oblique.

Part Position
• Rotate patient 35 to 45 degrees either right or left side up.
• Flex knee for stability.
• Center body to midline of grid.
• Adjust center of IR at level of iliac crests.
• Shield gonads.

Respiration:
Suspended expiration.

Central Ray
• Perpendicular to IR, entering elevated side 1 to 2 inches (2.5 to 5 cm) lateral to midline of body on elevated side and at level of iliac crests.

Collimation:
Adjust to 14 × 17 inches (35 × 43 cm). Place side marker in the collimated exposure field.

kVp: 120

Reference: 14th edition ATLAS p. 2:253.

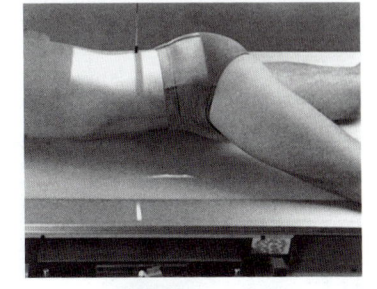

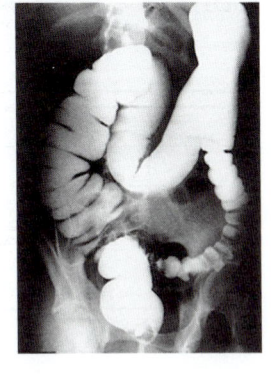

Manual Factors

Part Thickness (cm)	mA	kVp	Time	mAs	SID	Image Receptor Size	CR, DR Exposure Indicator	Grid	HF, 1Ø or 3Ø

AEC Factors

Part Thickness (cm)	mA	kVp	AEC Detector	mAs	Density Comp.	Image Receptor Size	CR, DR Exposure Indicator	Grid	HF, 1Ø or 3Ø

Notes: _____ Competency: ____/____/____

_____ Instructor: _____

Abdomen

Large Intestine
Lateral

Patient Position
• Position patient in lateral recumbent position.

Part Position
• Adjust body to true lateral position (right or left side down).
• Center midcoronal plane of abdomen to center of grid.
• Center IR to ASIS.
• Have patient flex knees and hips slightly and bring arms forward.
• Shield gonads.

Respiration:
Suspend.

Central Ray
• Perpendicular to IR, entering midcoronal plane at level of ASIS.

Collimation:
Adjust to 10 × 12 inches (24 × 30 cm). Place side marker in the collimated exposure field.

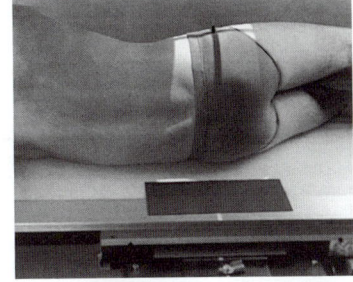

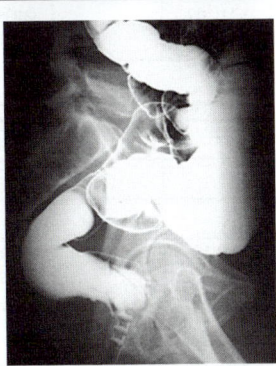

kVp: 120   *Reference: 14th edition ATLAS p. 2:255.*

Manual Factors

Part Thickness (cm)	mA	kVp	Time	mAs	SID	Image Receptor Size	CR, DR Exposure Indicator	Grid	HF, 1Ø or 3Ø

AEC Factors

Part Thickness (cm)	mA	kVp	AEC Detector	mAs	Density Comp.	Image Receptor Size	CR, DR Exposure Indicator	Grid	HF, 1Ø or 3Ø

Notes: _____ Competency: ____/____/____

_____ Instructor: _____

Abdomen

Large Intestine
AP

Patient Position
- Position patient supine.

Part Position
- Center midsagittal plane to grid.
- Center IR at level of iliac crests.
- Shield gonads.

Respiration:
Suspend.

Central Ray
- Perpendicular to IR, entering midsagittal plane at level of iliac crests.

Collimation:
Adjust to 14 × 17 inches (35 × 43 cm). Place side marker in the
collimated exposure field.

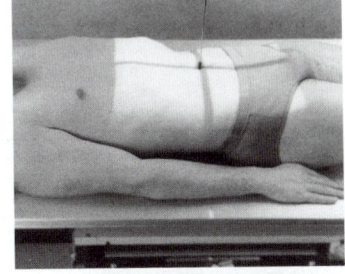
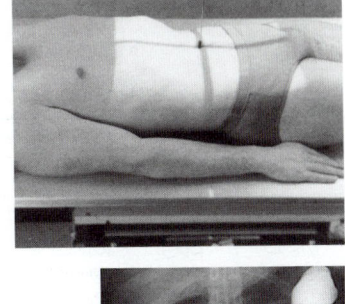
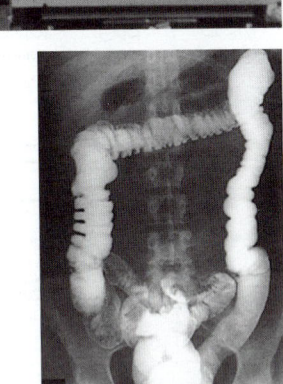

kVp: 120

Reference: 14th edition ATLAS p. 2:256.

Manual Factors

Part Thickness (cm)	mA	kVp	Time	mAs	SID	Image Receptor Size	CR, DR Exposure Indicator	Grid	HF, 1Ø or 3Ø

AEC Factors

Part Thickness (cm)	mA	kVp	AEC Detector	mAs	Density Comp.	Image Receptor Size	CR, DR Exposure Indicator	Grid	HF, 1Ø or 3Ø

Notes: _____ Competency: _____/___/___

Instructor: _____

Abdomen

Large Intestine
AP axial

Patient Position
• Position patient supine.

Part Position
• Center midsagittal plane to grid.
• Center IR 2 inches (5 cm) above iliac crests.
• Shield gonads.

Respiration:
Suspend.

Central Ray
• Angle 30 to 40 degrees cephalad, entering approximately 2 inches (5 cm) below level of ASIS. (When retrosigmoid is of interest, central ray enters inferior margin of pubic symphysis.)

Collimation:
Adjust to 14 × 17 inches (35 × 43 cm). Place side marker in the collimated exposure field.

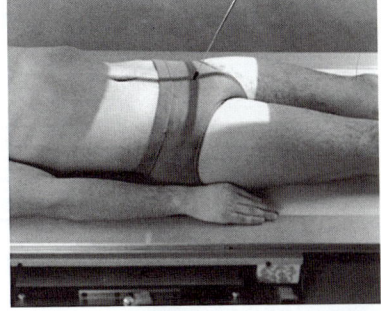

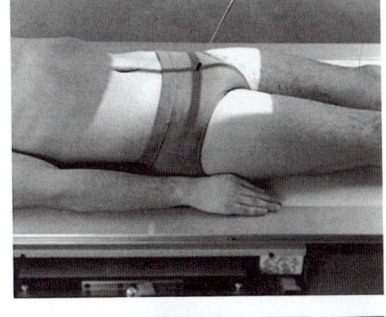

kVp: 120
Reference: 14th edition ATLAS p. 2:257.

Manual Factors

Part Thickness (cm)	mA	kVp	Time	mAs	SID	Image Receptor Size	CR, DR Exposure Indicator	Grid	HF, 1Ø or 3Ø

AEC Factors

Part Thickness (cm)	mA	kVp	AEC Detector	mAs	Density Comp.	Image Receptor Size	CR, DR Exposure Indicator	Grid	HF, 1Ø or 3Ø

Notes: _____ Competency: ____/____/____

Instructor: _____

Abdomen

Large Intestine
AP oblique (LPO and RPO)

Patient Position
• Position patient AP oblique.

Part Position
• Rotate patient 35 to 45 degrees from AP position either right or left side up.
• Center abdomen to grid.
• Adjust center of IR to level of iliac crests.
• Shield gonads.

Respiration:
Suspend.

Central Ray
• Perpendicular, entering elevated side 1 to 2 inches (2.5 to 5 cm) lateral to midline of body at level of iliac crests.

Collimation:
Adjust to 14 × 17 inches (35 × 43 cm). Place side marker in the collimated exposure field.

kVp: 120   *Reference: 14th edition ATLAS pp. 2:258-259.*

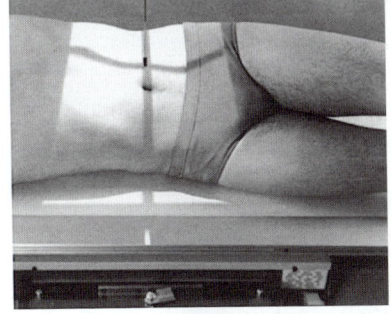
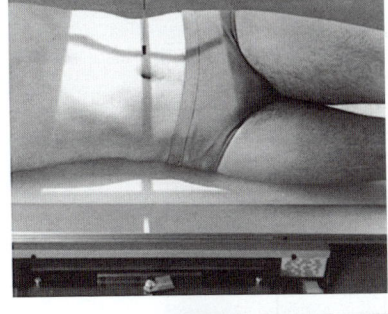

Manual Factors

Part Thickness (cm)	mA	kVp	Time	mAs	SID	Image Receptor Size	CR, DR Exposure Indicator	Grid	HF, 1Ø or 3Ø

AEC Factors

Part Thickness (cm)	mA	kVp	AEC Detector	mAs	Density Comp.	Image Receptor Size	CR, DR Exposure Indicator	Grid	HF, 1Ø or 3Ø

Notes: _____ Competency: ____/____/____

_____ Instructor: _____

Abdomen

Large Intestine
AP or PA (lateral decubitus)

Patient Position
• Position patient recumbent on either right or left side.
• Elevate dependent side on firm pad.

Part Position
• Place arms above head, with knees slightly flexed.
• Center midsagittal plane to grid.
• Center IR to midsagittal plane at level of iliac crests.
• Shield gonads.

Respiration:
Suspend.

Central Ray
• Horizontal and perpendicular to IR at level of iliac crests.

Collimation:
Adjust to 14 × 17 inches (35 × 43 cm). Place side marker in the collimated exposure field.

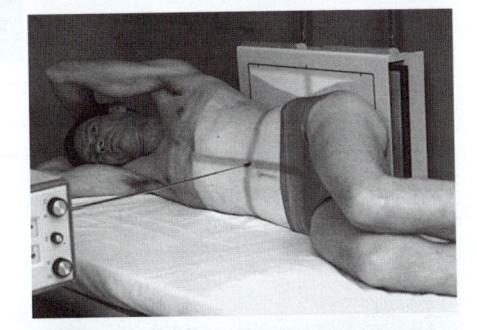

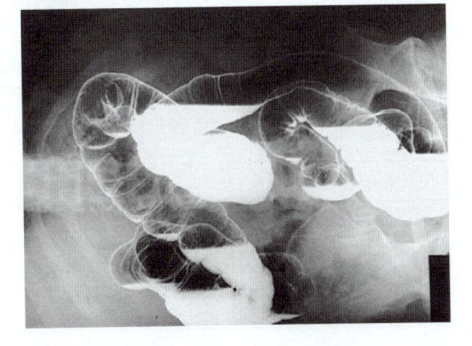

kVp: 120

Reference: 14th edition ATLAS p. 2:261.

Manual Factors

Part Thickness (cm)	mA	kVp	Time	mAs	SID	Image Receptor Size	CR, DR Exposure Indicator	Grid	HF, 1Ø or 3Ø

AEC Factors

Part Thickness (cm)	mA	kVp	AEC Detector	mAs	Density Comp.	Image Receptor Size	CR, DR Exposure Indicator	Grid	HF, 1Ø or 3Ø

Notes: _____ Competency: _____/____/____

_____ Instructor: _____

Abdomen

Large Intestine
Lateral, AP or PA oblique (upright)

Patient Position
• Position patient upright—frontal, lateral, or oblique.

Part Position
• Adjust arms to remove from area of interest, and distribute weight equally on feet.
• Center IR at level of iliac crests and (1) midsagittal plane for AP or PA projection, (2) midway between midsagittal plane and lateral aspect of side of interest for oblique positions, or (3) midcoronal plane for lateral position.
• Shield gonads.

Respiration:
Suspend.

Central Ray
• Perpendicular to IR at *level of iliac crests.*

Collimation:
Adjust to 14 × 17 inches (35 × 43 cm). Place side marker in the collimated exposure field.

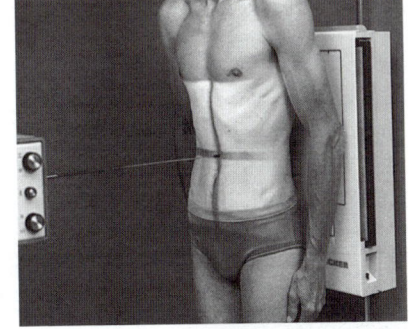

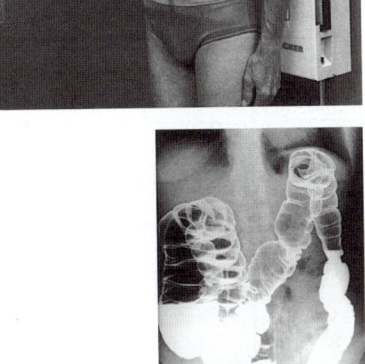

kVp: 120   *Reference: 14th edition ATLAS p. 2:266.*

Manual Factors

Part Thickness (cm)	mA	kVp	Time	mAs	SID	Image Receptor Size	CR, DR Exposure Indicator	Grid	HF, 1Ø or 3Ø

AEC Factors

Part Thickness (cm)	mA	kVp	AEC Detector	mAs	Density Comp.	Image Receptor Size	CR, DR Exposure Indicator	Grid	HF, 1Ø or 3Ø

Notes: _____ Competency: ____/____/____

Instructor: _____

Abdomen

Urinary System
AP oblique (RPO and LPO)

Patient Position
• Position patient supine.

Part Position
• Rotate patient 30 degrees from IR plane.
• Place support under elevated side as needed.
• Adjust hips and shoulders to be in same planes.
• Center spine to grid.
• Center IR at level of iliac crests.
• Shield gonads.

Respiration:
Suspend.

Central Ray
• Perpendicular to level of iliac crests, entering elevated side approximately 2 inches (5 cm) lateral to midline.

NOTE: For AP, PA, lateral, and decubitus positioning for the urinary system, see similar abdomen positions in this section.

Collimation:
Adjust to 14 × 17 inches (35 × 43 cm). Place side marker in the collimated exposure field.

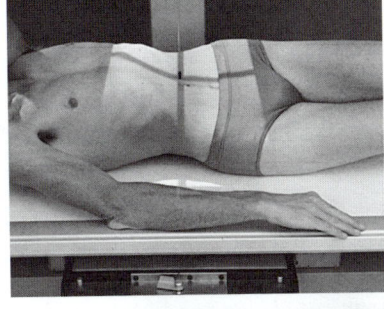

kVp: 80   Reference: 14th edition ATLAS p. 2-306

Manual Factors

Part Thickness (cm)	mA	kVp	Time	mAs	SID	Image Receptor Size	CR, DR Exposure Indicator	Grid	HF, 1Ø or 3Ø

AEC Factors

Part Thickness (cm)	mA	kVp	AEC Detector	mAs	Density Comp.	Image Receptor Size	CR, DR Exposure Indicator	Grid	HF, 1Ø or 3Ø

Notes: _____ Competency: _____/_____/_____

_____ Instructor: _____

Abdomen

Bladder
AP or PA axial

Patient Position
• Position patient supine.

Part Position
• Center midsagittal plane to grid (1) 2 to 3 inches (5 to 7.5 cm) above pubic symphysis to show the bladder or (2) at pubic symphysis for voiding studies.
• Adjust shoulders and hips to be equidistant from IR.
• Have patient place arms across upper chest or at sides.
• Have patient extend legs.

Respiration:
Suspend.

Central Ray
• Adjust 10 to 15 degrees caudad (1) at level 2 to 3 inches (5 to 7.5 cm) above pubic symphysis to show bladder or (2) at pubic symphysis for voiding studies.

Collimation:
Adjust to 10 × 12 inches (24 × 30 cm). Place side marker in the collimated exposure field.

kVp: 80

Reference: 14th edition ATLAS p. 2:316.

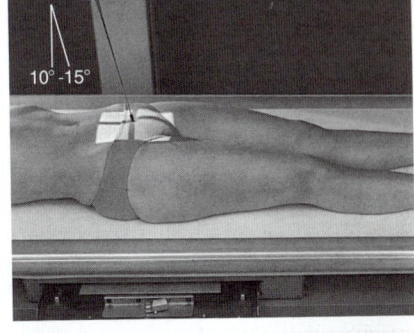
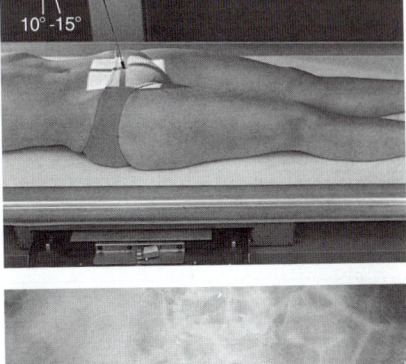

Manual Factors									
Part Thickness (cm)	mA	kVp	Time	mAs	SID	Image Receptor Size	CR, DR Exposure Indicator	Grid	HF, 1Ø or 3Ø

AEC Factors									
Part Thickness (cm)	mA	kVp	AEC Detector	mAs	Density Comp.	Image Receptor Size	CR, DR Exposure Indicator	Grid	HF, 1Ø or 3Ø

Notes: _____ Competency: ____/____/____

_____ Instructor: _____

Abdomen

Bladder
AP oblique (RPO or LPO)

Patient Position
• Position patient supine.

Part Position
• Rotate patient 40 to 60 degrees from supine.
• Center IR 2 to 3 inches (5 to 7.5 cm) above upper border of pubic symphysis and 2 inches (5 cm) medial to ASIS.
• Have patient abduct uppermost thigh to prevent its superimposition on bladder area.

Respiration:
Suspend.

Central Ray
• Perpendicular, entering elevated side 2 inches (5 cm) medial to midsagittal plane (1) at 2 to 3 inches (5 to 7.5 cm) superior to pubic symphysis or (2) at pubic symphysis for voiding studies.
NOTE: RPO position is also used for male cystourethrography.

Collimation:
Adjust to 10 × 12 inches (24 × 30 cm). Place side marker in the collimated exposure field.

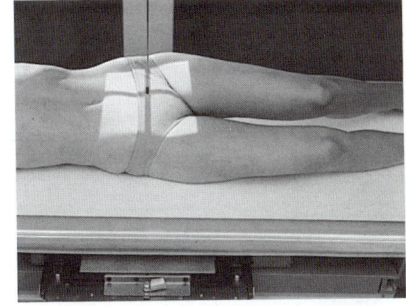
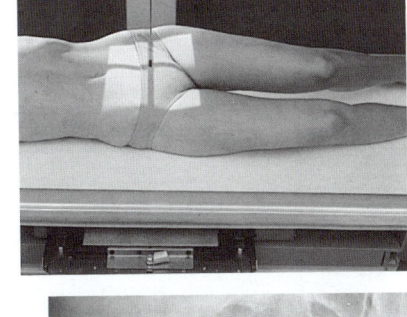

kVp: 80   *Reference: 14th edition ATLAS p. 2:318.*

Manual Factors

Part Thickness (cm)	mA	kVp	Time	mAs	SID	Image Receptor Size	CR, DR Exposure Indicator	Grid	HF, 1Ø or 3Ø

AEC Factors

Part Thickness (cm)	mA	kVp	AEC Detector	mAs	Density Comp.	Image Receptor Size	CR, DR Exposure Indicator	Grid	HF, 1Ø or 3Ø

Notes: _____ Competency: ____/____/____

Instructor: _____

Abdomen

Bladder
Lateral

Patient Position
• Position patient lateral recumbent (either left or right).

Part Position
• Center midcoronal plane to grid.
• Have patient flex hips and knees.
• Adjust patient's arms forward with hands under head.
• Center IR 2 inches (5 cm) above pubic symphysis.

Respiration:
Suspend.

Central Ray
• Perpendicular to IR, entering 2 inches (5 cm) above pubic symphysis.

Collimation:
Adjust to 10 × 12 inches (24 × 30 cm). Place side marker in the collimated exposure field.

kVp: 85   *Reference: 14th edition ATLAS p. 2:320.*

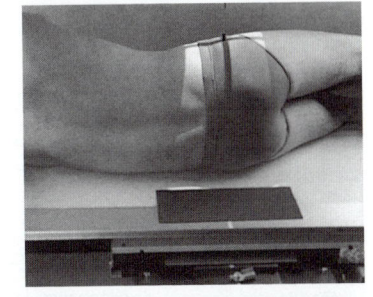

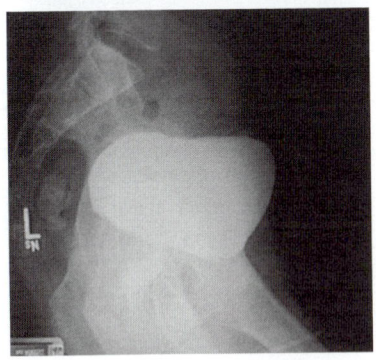

Manual Factors

Part Thickness (cm)	mA	kVp	Time	mAs	SID	Image Receptor Size	CR, DR Exposure Indicator	Grid	HF, 1Ø or 3Ø

AEC Factors

Part Thickness (cm)	mA	kVp	AEC Detector	mAs	Density Comp.	Image Receptor Size	CR, DR Exposure Indicator	Grid	HF, 1Ø or 3Ø

Notes: _____ Competency: _____/_____/_____

_____ Instructor: _____

Abdomen

Cranial Lines, Planes, and Abbreviations, 272

Cranium:
PA and PA axial; CALDWELL METHOD, 274
AP and AP axial, 276
Lateral, 278
AP axial; TOWNE METHOD, 280
PA axial; HAAS METHOD, 282
Submentovertical; SCHÜLLER METHOD, 284

Facial Bones:
Lateral, 286
Parietoacanthial; WATERS METHOD, 288
Acanthoparietal; REVERSE WATERS METHOD, 290

Nasal Bones:
Lateral, 292

Zygomatic Arches:
Submentovertical, 294

Zygomatic Arches:
Tangential, 296

Zygomatic Arches:
AP axial; MODIFIED TOWNE METHOD, 298

Mandibular Rami:
PA, 300
PA axial, 302

Mandible:
Axiolateral and axiolateral oblique, 304

Temporomandibular Articulations:
AP axial, 306

Temporomandibular Articulations:
Axiolateral oblique, 308

Paranasal Sinuses:
Lateral, 310

Frontal and Anterior Ethmoidal Sinuses:
PA axial; CALDWELL METHOD, 312

Maxillary Sinuses:
Parietoacanthial; WATERS METHOD, 314

Ethmoidal and Sphenoidal Sinuses:
Submentovertical, 316

Cranial Lines, Planes, and Abbreviations

Abbreviations Used in This Section

AML: acanthomeatal line
EAM: external acoustic meatus
IOML: infraorbitomeatal line
OML: orbitomeatal line

- Glabella
- Midsagittal plane
- Interpupillary line
- Inner canthus
- Nasion
- Acanthion
- Mental point
- Angle of mandible (gonion)
- Infraorbital margin
- Outer canthus

Reference: 14th edition ATLAS p. 2:29.

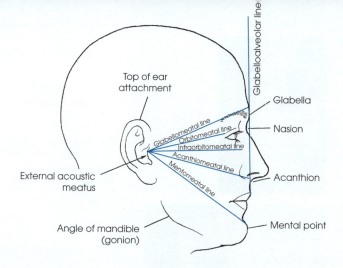

Cranium

Cranium
PA and PA axial CALDWELL METHOD

Patient Position
• Position patient seated upright or prone.

Part Position
• Have patient rest head on forehead and nose.
• Position midsagittal plane perpendicular to midline of grid device.
• OML is perpendicular to IR.

Respiration:
Suspend.

Central Ray
• *PA:* Perpendicular to IR, exiting nasion.
• *Caldwell method:* Angle 15 degrees caudad, exiting nasion.
• Center IR to central ray.

Collimation:
Adjust radiation field to extend ½ to 1 inch (1.3 to 2.5 cm) beyond the
skin line of the skull. Check for light at vertex and on both sides.
Place side marker in the collimated exposure field.

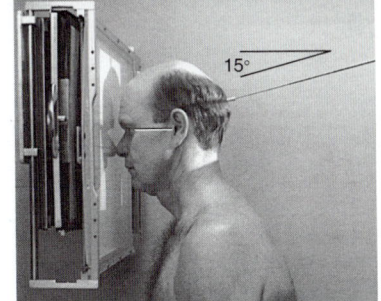

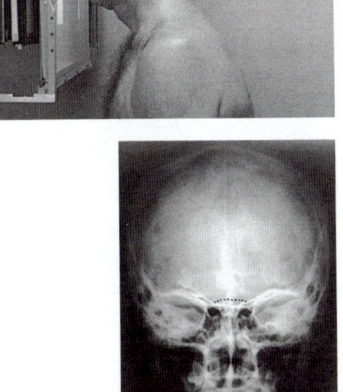

kVp: 85

Reference: 14th edition ATLAS p. 2:38.

Manual Factors

Part Thickness (cm)	mA	kVp	Time	mAs	SID	Image Receptor Size	CR, DR Exposure Indicator	Grid	HF, 1Ø or 3Ø

AEC Factors

Part Thickness (cm)	mA	kVp	AEC Detector	mAs	Density Comp.	Image Receptor Size	CR, DR Exposure Indicator	Grid	HF, 1Ø or 3Ø

Notes: _____ Competency: ____/____/____

_____ Instructor: _____

Cranium

Cranium
AP and AP axial

Patient Position
• Position patient supine.

Part Position
• Position midsagittal plane and OML perpendicular to IR.
• Place arms at sides or across chest.

Respiration:
Suspend.

Central Ray
• *AP:* Perpendicular to nasion.
• *AP axial:* Angle 15 degrees cephalad.
• Center IR to central ray.

Collimation:
Adjust radiation field to extend ½ to 1 inch (1.3 to 2.5 cm) beyond the skin line of the skull. Check for light at vertex and on both sides. Place side marker in the collimated exposure field.

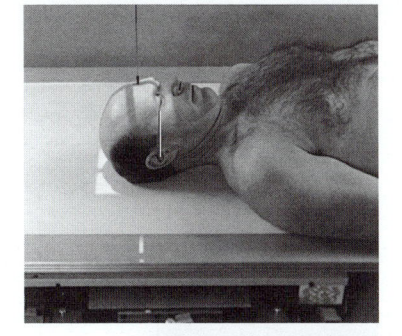

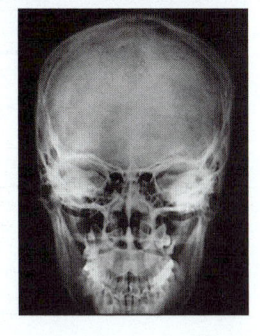

kVp: 85

Reference: 14th edition ATLAS p. 2:42.

Manual Factors

Part Thickness (cm)	mA	kVp	Time	mAs	SID	Image Receptor Size	CR, DR Exposure Indicator	Grid	HF, 1Ø or 3Ø

AEC Factors

Part Thickness (cm)	mA	kVp	AEC Detector	mAs	Density Comp.	Image Receptor Size	CR, DR Exposure Indicator	Grid	HF, 1Ø or 3Ø

Notes: _____ Competency: _____/_____/_____

_____ Instructor: _____

Cranium

Cranium
Lateral

Patient Position
• Position patient seated upright or semiprone.

Part Position
• Position midsagittal plane parallel to IR.
• IOML is perpendicular to front edge of IR.
• Interpupillary line is perpendicular to IR.

Respiration:
Suspend.

Central Ray
• Perpendicular entering 2 inches (5 cm) superior to EAM.
• Center IR to central ray.

Collimation:
Adjust radiation field to extend ½ to 1 inch (1.3 to 2.5 cm) beyond the skin line of the skull. Check for light at vertex, anterior, posterior, and base of the skull borders. Place side marker in the collimated exposure field.

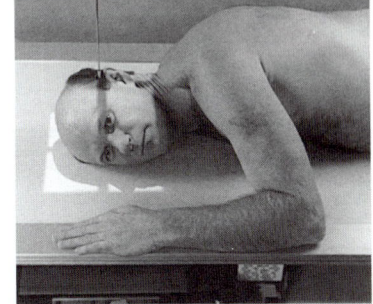

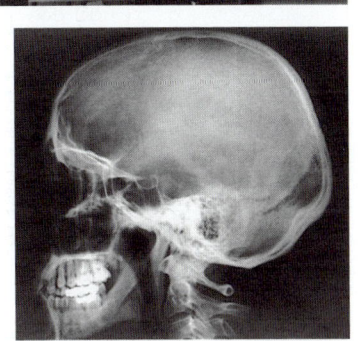

kVp: 85

Reference: 14th edition ATLAS p. 2:34.

Manual Factors

Part Thickness (cm)	mA	kVp	Time	mAs	SID	Image Receptor Size	CR, DR Exposure Indicator	Grid	HF, 1Ø or 3Ø

AEC Factors

Part Thickness (cm)	mA	kVp	AEC Detector	mAs	Density Comp.	Image Receptor Size	CR, DR Exposure Indicator	Grid	HF, 1Ø or 3Ø

Notes: _____ Competency: _____/____/____

_____ Instructor: _____

Cranium

Cranium
AP axial TOWNE METHOD

Patient Position
• Position patient seated upright or supine.

Part Position
• Center midsagittal plane to midline of grid device, and adjust to make perpendicular.
• Have patient flex neck, and adjust OML perpendicular to IR.
• When patient cannot flex neck, place IOML perpendicular.
• Place top of IR at level of cranial vertex.

Respiration:
Suspend.

Central Ray
• Direct through foramen magnum with caudal angle of 30 degrees to OML or 37 degrees to IOML. Central ray enters approximately 2 ½ inches (6.4 cm) superior to glabella and passes through level of EAM.

Collimation:
Adjust the radiation field to extend ½ to 1 inch (1.3 to 2.5 cm) beyond the skin line of the skull. Check for light at the vertex and on both sides. Place side marker in the collimated exposure field.

kVp: 85

Reference: 14th edition ATLAS p. 2:44.

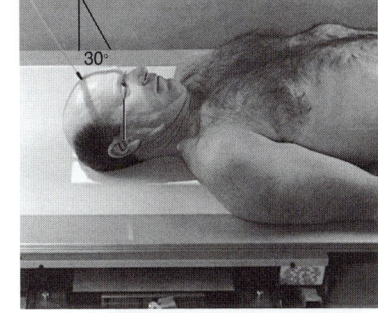

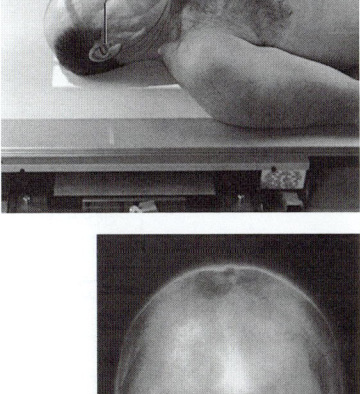

Manual Factors

Part Thickness (cm)	mA	kVp	Time	mAs	SID	Image Receptor Size	CR, DR Exposure Indicator	Grid	HF, 1Ø or 3Ø

AEC Factors

Part Thickness (cm)	mA	kVp	AEC Detector	mAs	Density Comp.	Image Receptor Size	CR, DR Exposure Indicator	Grid	HF, 1Ø or 3Ø

Notes: _____ Competency: ____/____/____

_____ Instructor: _____

Cranium

Cranium
PA axial HAAS METHOD

Patient Position
• Position patient seated upright or prone.

Part Position
• Have patient rest head on forehead and nose.
• Place arms in comfortable position.
• Adjust shoulders to lie in same transverse plane.
• Adjust head so that midsagittal plane and OML are perpendicular to IR.

Respiration:
Suspend.

Central Ray
• Direct 25 degrees cephalad, entering 1½ inches (3.8 cm) inferior to external occipital protuberance (inion) and exiting 1½ inches (3.8 cm) superior to nasion.

Collimation:
Adjust the radiation field to extend ½ to 1 inch (1.3 to 2.5 cm) beyond the skin line of the skull. Check for light at the vertex and on both sides. Place side marker in the collimated exposure field.

kVp: 85

Reference: 14th edition ATLAS p. 2:50.

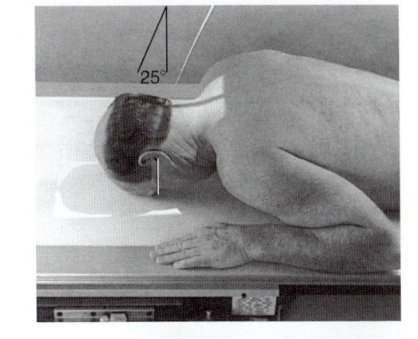

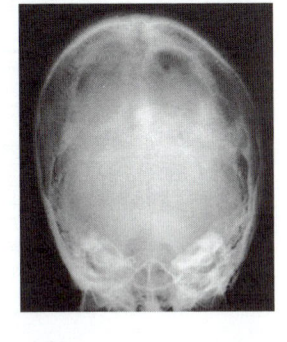

Manual Factors

Part Thickness (cm)	mA	kVp	Time	mAs	SID	Image Receptor Size	CR, DR Exposure Indicator	Grid	HF, 1Ø or 3Ø

AEC Factors

Part Thickness (cm)	mA	kVp	AEC Detector	mAs	Density Comp.	Image Receptor Size	CR, DR Exposure Indicator	Grid	HF, 1Ø or 3Ø

Notes: _____ Competency: _____/___/___

_____ Instructor: _____

Cranium

Cranium
Submentovertical SCHÜLLER METHOD

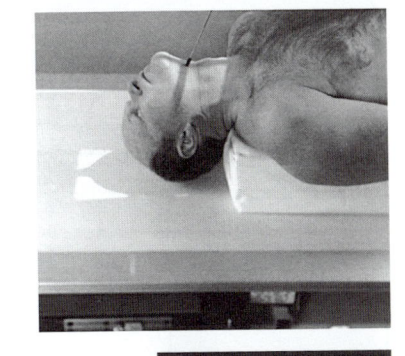

Patient Position
• Position patient seated upright at head unit or supine on elevated table support.

Part Position
• Have patient extend neck and rest head on vertex.
• Center and adjust midsagittal plane perpendicular to IR.
• Adjust IOML parallel to plane of IR if possible.
• Immobilize head.

Respiration:
Suspend.

Central Ray
• Direct through sella turcica perpendicular to IOML entering between angles of mandible.
• Central ray passes through a point ¾ inch (1.9 cm) anterior to level of EAM.

Collimation:
Adjust the radiation field to extend ½ inch (1.3 cm) beyond the shadow of the tip of the nose and 1 inch beyond the lateral borders. Place side marker in the collimated exposure field.

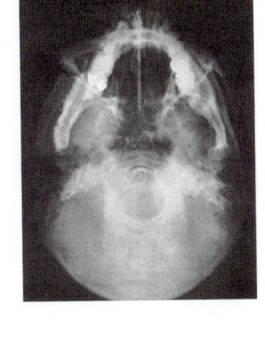

kVp: 85

Reference: 14th edition ATLAS p. 2-52

Manual Factors

Part Thickness (cm)	mA	kVp	Time	mAs	SID	Image Receptor Size	CR, DR Exposure Indicator	Grid	HF, 1Ø or 3Ø

AEC Factors

Part Thickness (cm)	mA	kVp	AEC Detector	mAs	Density Comp.	Image Receptor Size	CR, DR Exposure Indicator	Grid	HF, 1Ø or 3Ø

Notes: _____ Competency: ____/____/____

_____ Instructor: _____

Cranium

Facial Bones
Lateral

Patient Position
- Position patient seated upright or semiprone.

Part Position
- Position zygomatic bone to center of grid.
- Adjust midsagittal plane parallel to IR.
- IOML is parallel to transverse axis of IR.
- Interpupillary line is perpendicular to IR.

Respiration
Suspend.

Central Ray
- Perpendicular entering lateral surface of zygomatic bone halfway between outer canthus and EAM.
- Center IR to central ray.

Collimation:
Adjust to extend ½ inch (1.3 cm) beyond the shadow of the tip of the nose, superiorly to ½ inch (1.3 cm) above the supraorbital margins, inferiorly to the gonion, and posteriorly to the EAM. The exposure field should be set no larger than 6 × 10 inches (15 × 24 cm). Place side marker in the collimated exposure field.

kVp: 80

Reference: 14th edition ATLAS p. 2-62

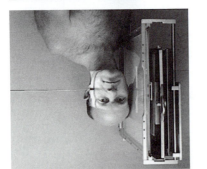
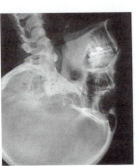

Manual Factors

Part Thickness (cm)	mA	kVp	Time	mAs	SID	Image Receptor Size	CR, DR Exposure Indicator	Grid	HF, 1Ø or 3Ø

AEC Factors

Part Thickness (cm)	mA	kVp	AEC Detector	mAs	Density Comp.	Image Receptor Size	CR, DR Exposure Indicator	Grid	HF, 1Ø or 3Ø

Notes: _____ Competency: _____/_____/_____

_____ Instructor: _____

Cranium

Facial Bones
Parietoacanthial   WATERS METHOD

Patient Position
• Position patient seated upright or prone.

Part Position
• Center and adjust midsagittal plane perpendicular to IR, and have patient rest head on extended chin.
• Hyperextend neck and adjust OML to form 37-degree angle to IR plane.
• Mentomeatal line is approximately perpendicular to IR.
• Usually patient's nose is about ¾ inch (1.9 cm) from grid device.
• Center IR to acanthion.

Respiration:
Suspend.

Central Ray
• Perpendicular, exiting acanthion.

Collimation:
Adjust to ½ to 1 inch (1.3 to 2.5 cm) beyond the shadows of the lateral sides of the face, superiorly to include the supraorbital margins and inferiorly to the level of the chin. The exposure field should be no larger than 8 × 10 inches (18 × 24 cm). Place side marker in the collimated exposure field.

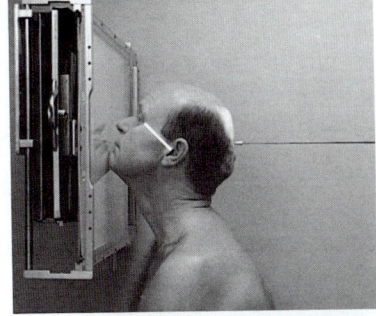

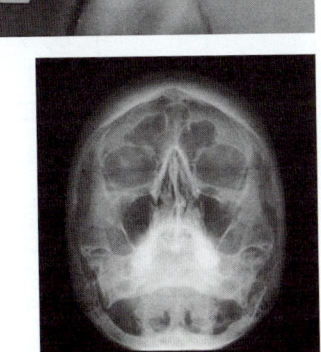

Manual Factors

Part Thickness (cm)	mA	kVp	Time	mAs	SID	Image Receptor Size	CR, DR Exposure Indicator	Grid	HF, 1Ø or 3Ø

AEC Factors

Part Thickness (cm)	mA	kVp	AEC Detector	mAs	Density Comp.	Image Receptor Size	CR, DR Exposure Indicator	Grid	HF, 1Ø or 3Ø

Notes: _____ Competency: ____/____/____

Instructor: _____

Cranium

Facial Bones
Acanthoparietal REVERSE WATERS METHOD

Patient Position
• Position patient supine.

Part Position
• Center and adjust midsagittal plane perpendicular to IR.
• Adjust extension of neck so that OML forms 37-degree angle with plane of IR. If necessary, place a support under patient's shoulders to help extend the neck.
• Mentomeatal line is approximately perpendicular to plane of IR.
• Adjust head so that midsagittal plane is perpendicular to plane of IR.

Respiration:
Suspend.

Central Ray
• Perpendicular to enter acanthion.
• Center IR to central ray.

Collimation:
Adjust to extend about ½ to 1 inch (1.3 to 2.5 cm) beyond the lateral sides of the face, superiorly just to the skin shadow, and inferiorly to the chin. The exposure field should be no larger than 8 × 10 inches (18 × 24 cm). Place side marker in the collimated exposure field.

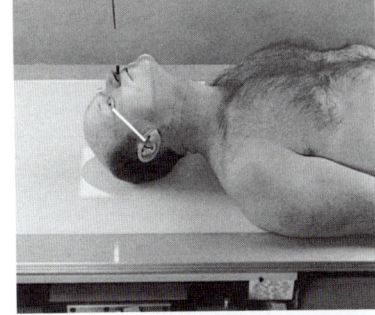
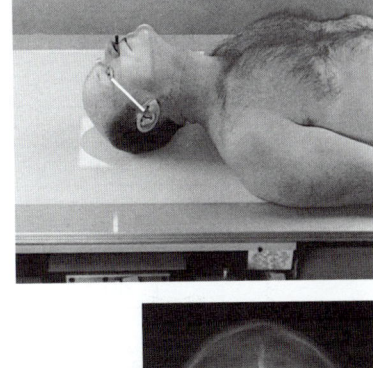

Manual Factors

Part Thickness (cm)	mA	kVp	Time	mAs	SID	Image Receptor Size	CR, DR Exposure Indicator	Grid	HF, 1Ø or 3Ø

AEC Factors

Part Thickness (cm)	mA	kVp	AEC Detector	mAs	Density Comp.	Image Receptor Size	CR, DR Exposure Indicator	Grid	HF, 1Ø or 3Ø

Notes: _____ Competency: _____/_____/_____

_____ Instructor: _____

Cranium

Nasal Bones
Lateral

Patient Position
• Position patient seated upright or semiprone.

Part Position
• Center nasion to IR.
• Adjust midsagittal plane parallel to IR.
• IOML is parallel to transverse axis of IR.
• Interpupillary line is perpendicular to IR.

Respiration:
Suspend.

Central Ray
• Perpendicular, entering ½ inch (1.3 cm) distal to nasion.
• Ensure that collimation is extremely close.

Collimation:
Adjust to extend from the glabella to 1 inch (2.5 cm) inferior to the acanthion and ½ inch (1.3 cm) beyond the tip of the nose. The exposure field should be no larger than 3 × 3 inches (8 × 8 cm). Place side marker in the collimated exposure field.

kVp: 70

Reference: 14th edition ATLAS p. 2:73.

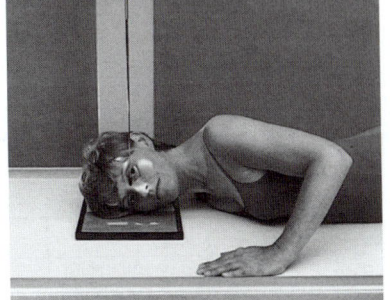

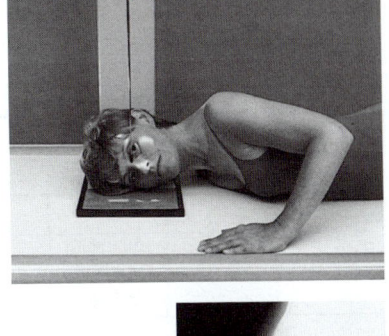

Manual Factors

Part Thickness (cm)	mA	kVp	Time	mAs	SID	Image Receptor Size	CR, DR Exposure Indicator	Grid	HF, 1Ø or 3Ø

AEC Factors

Part Thickness (cm)	mA	kVp	AEC Detector	mAs	Density Comp.	Image Receptor Size	CR, DR Exposure Indicator	Grid	HF, 1Ø or 3Ø

Notes: _____ Competency: ____/____/____

_____ Instructor: _____

Cranium

Zygomatic Arches
Submentovertical

Patient Position
• Position patient seated upright or supine on elevated table support.

Part Position
• Hyperextend neck, and have patient rest head on vertex.
• Center and adjust midsagittal plane perpendicular to IR.
• Adjust IOML parallel to IR if possible.

Respiration:
Suspend.

Central Ray
• Perpendicular to IOML, entering midway between zygomatic arches.
• Central ray enters approximately 1 inch (2.5 cm) posterior to outer canthi.

Collimation:
Adjust to extend ½ to 1 inch (1.3 to 2.5 cm) beyond the lateral sides of the face, superiorly to the chin, and inferiorly to the gonions. The exposure field should be no larger than 8 × 10 inches (18 × 24 cm). Place side marker in the collimated exposure field.

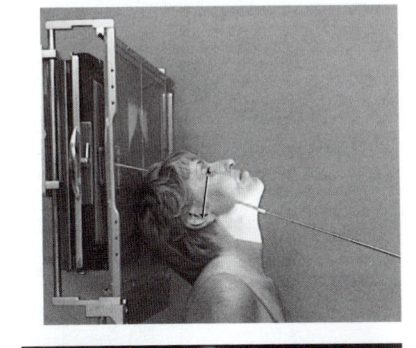

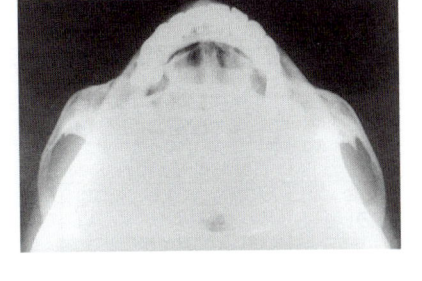

kVp: 80

Reference: 14th edition ATLAS p. 2:75.

Manual Factors

Part Thickness (cm)	mA	kVp	Time	mAs	SID	Image Receptor Size	CR, DR Exposure Indicator	Grid	HF, 1Ø or 3Ø

AEC Factors

Part Thickness (cm)	mA	kVp	AEC Detector	mAs	Density Comp.	Image Receptor Size	CR, DR Exposure Indicator	Grid	HF, 1Ø or 3Ø

Notes: _____ Competency: _____/_____/_____

_____ Instructor: _____

Cranium

Zygomatic Arches
Tangential

Patient Position
• Position patient seated upright or supine on elevated table support.

Part Position
• Hyperextend neck, and have patient rest head on vertex.
• Center zygomatic arch and adjust midsagittal plane perpendicular to IR.
• Adjust IOML as parallel as possible to IR.
• Rotate midsagittal plane 15 degrees toward side being examined, then tilt top of head approximately 15 degrees away from side being examined so that central ray is tangent to zygomatic arch.

Respiration:
Suspend.

Central Ray
• Perpendicular to IOML, entering affected zygomatic arch at a point 1 inch (2.5 cm) posterior to outer canthus

Collimation:
Adjust to ½ inch (1.3 cm) beyond the skin shadow of the affected cheek, superiorly to the tip of the nose, and inferiorly to the gonion. The exposure field should be no larger than 6 × 10 inches (18 × 24 cm). Place side marker in the collimated exposure field.

kVp: 80   *Reference: 14th edition ATLAS p. 2-77*

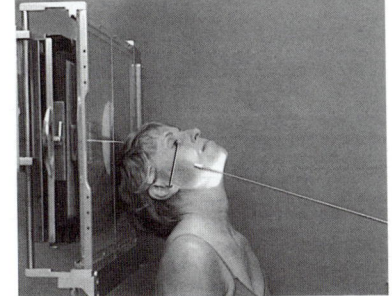

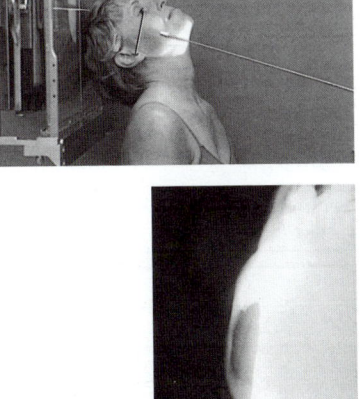

Manual Factors

Part Thickness (cm)	mA	kVp	Time	mAs	SID	Image Receptor Size	CR, DR Exposure Indicator	Grid	HF, 1Ø or 3Ø

AEC Factors

Part Thickness (cm)	mA	kVp	AEC Detector	mAs	Density Comp.	Image Receptor Size	CR, DR Exposure Indicator	Grid	HF, 1Ø or 3Ø

Notes: _____ Competency: ____/____/____

Instructor: _____

Cranium

Zygomatic Arches
AP axial   MODIFIED TOWNE METHOD

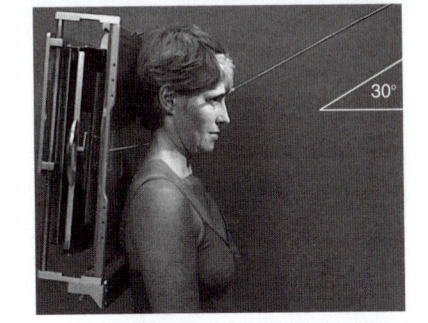

Patient Position
• Position patient seated upright or supine.

Part Position
• Center midsagittal plane to grid device, and adjust to perpendicular position.
• Flex neck, and adjust OML perpendicular to IR.

Respiration:
Suspend.

Central Ray
• Angle 30 degrees caudad, entering glabella approximately 1 inch (2.5 cm) superior to nasion. (Direct 37 degrees caudad if IOML is perpendicular to IR.)
• Center IR to central ray.

Collimation:
Adjust to extend ½ to 1 inch (1.3 to 2.5 cm) beyond the lateral sides of the face, superiorly to the top of the forehead, and inferiorly to the chin. The exposure field should be no larger than 10 × 8 inches (24 × 18 cm). Place side marker in the collimated exposure field.

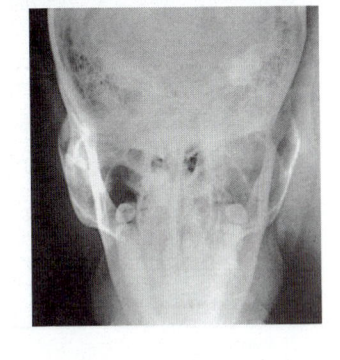

kVp: 80   *Reference: 14th edition ATLAS p. 2:79.*

Manual Factors

Part Thickness (cm)	mA	kVp	Time	mAs	SID	Image Receptor Size	CR, DR Exposure Indicator	Grid	HF, 1Ø or 3Ø

AEC Factors

Part Thickness (cm)	mA	kVp	AEC Detector	mAs	Density Comp.	Image Receptor Size	CR, DR Exposure Indicator	Grid	HF, 1Ø or 3Ø

Notes: _____ Competency: _____/___/___

_____ Instructor: _____

Cranium

Mandibular Rami
PA

Patient Position
• Position patient seated upright or prone.

Part Position
• Have patient rest forehead and nose on grid device.
• Adjust head so that midsagittal plane is perpendicular to IR.
• OML is perpendicular to IR.

Respiration:
Suspend.

Central Ray
• Perpendicular to exit acanthion.
• Center IR to central ray.

Collimation:
Adjust to extend ½ to 1 inch (1.3 to 2.5 cm) beyond the lateral sides, above the TMJs and below the chin. The exposure field should be no larger than 8 × 10 inches (18 × 24 cm). Place side marker in the collimated exposure field.

kVp: 80

Reference: 14th edition ATLAS p. 2:81.

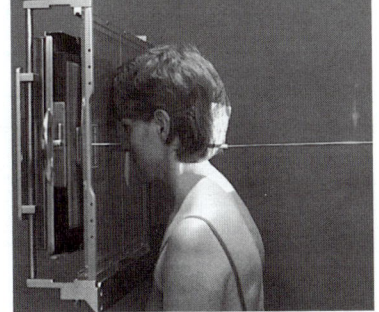
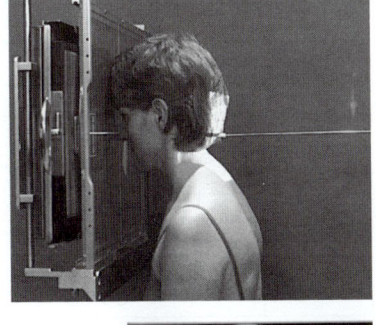

Manual Factors

Part Thickness (cm)	mA	kVp	Time	mAs	SID	Image Receptor Size	CR, DR Exposure Indicator	Grid	HF, 1Ø or 3Ø

AEC Factors

Part Thickness (cm)	mA	kVp	AEC Detector	mAs	Density Comp.	Image Receptor Size	CR, DR Exposure Indicator	Grid	HF, 1Ø or 3Ø

Notes: _____

Competency: ___/___/___

Instructor: _____

Cranium

Mandibular Rami
PA axial

Patient Position
• Position patient seated upright or prone.

Part Position
• Position midsagittal plane perpendicular to IR.
• OML is perpendicular to IR.
• Have patient rest forehead and nose on IR holder.

Respiration:
Suspend.

Central Ray
• Angle 20 to 25 degrees cephalad, exiting at acanthion.
• Center IR to central ray.

Collimation:
Adjust to extend ½ to 1 inch (1.3 to 2.5 cm) beyond the lateral sides, above the TMJs and below the chin. The exposure field should be no larger than 8 × 10 inches (18 × 24 cm). Place side marker in the collimated exposure field.

kVp: 80

Reference: 14th edition ATLAS p. 2:82.

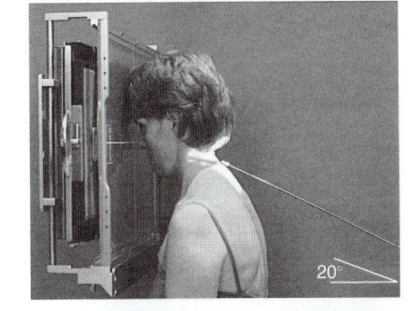

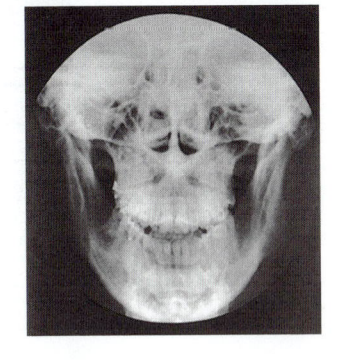

Manual Factors

Part Thickness (cm)	mA	kVp	Time	mAs	SID	Image Receptor Size	CR, DR Exposure Indicator	Grid	HF, 1Ø or 3Ø

AEC Factors

Part Thickness (cm)	mA	kVp	AEC Detector	mAs	Density Comp.	Image Receptor Size	CR, DR Exposure Indicator	Grid	HF, 1Ø or 3Ø

Notes: _____ Competency: _____/____/____

_____ Instructor: _____

Cranium

Mandible
Axiolateral and axiolateral oblique

Patient Position
- Position patient seated upright, semisupine, or semiprone.

Part Position
- Place head in lateral position with interpupillary line perpendicular.
- Extend neck enough that long axis of mandibular body is parallel to transverse axis of IR, preventing superimposition of cervical spine.
- If projection is being performed on tabletop, position IR so that complete body of mandible is positioned on IR.
- Adjust rotation of head so that area of interest is parallel to IR as follows: (1) for *ramus,* keep head in true lateral position; (2) for *body,* rotate head 30 degrees toward IR; (3) for *symphysis,* rotate head 45 degrees toward IR.

Respiration:
Suspend.

Central Ray
- Angle 25 degrees cephalad to pass directly through mandibular region of interest.

Collimation:
Adjust to extend ½ to 1 inch (1.3 to 2.5 cm) beyond the anterior and inferior skin shadows and above the TMJ. The exposure field should be no larger than 8 × 10 inches (18 × 24 cm). Place side marker in the collimated exposure field.

kVp: 80

Reference: 14th edition ATLAS p. 2-85

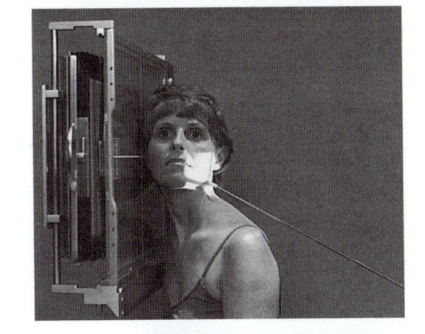

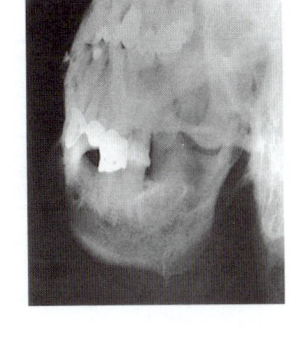

Manual Factors

Part Thickness (cm)	mA	kVp	Time	mAs	SID	Image Receptor Size	CR, DR Exposure Indicator	Grid	HF, 1Ø or 3Ø

AEC Factors

Part Thickness (cm)	mA	kVp	AEC Detector	mAs	Density Comp.	Image Receptor Size	CR, DR Exposure Indicator	Grid	HF, 1Ø or 3Ø

Notes: _____ Competency: ____/____/____

Instructor: _____

Cranium

Temporomandibular Articulations
AP axial

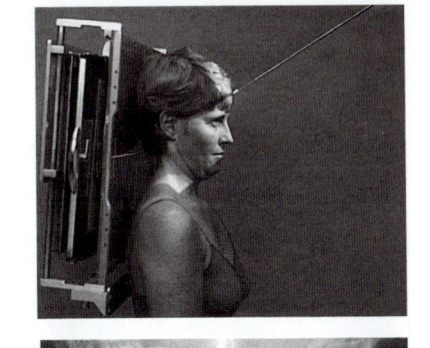

Patient Position
• Position patient seated upright or supine.

Part Position
• Adjust head so that midsagittal plane is perpendicular to IR.
• Flex neck to place OML perpendicular to IR.
• After first exposure with patient's mouth closed, do not permit patient to move. Change IR, and make second exposure with mouth fully open.

Respiration:
Suspend.

Central Ray
• Angle 35 degrees caudal, centered to temporomandibular joints and entering approximately 3 inches (7.6 cm) superior to nasion.
• Center IR to central ray.

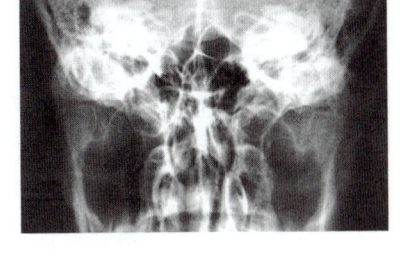

Collimation:
Adjust to extend ½ inch to 1 inch (1.3 to 2.5 cm) beyond the lateral sides, superiorly to the glabella, and inferiorly to the lips. The exposure field should be no larger than 8 × 10 inches (18 × 24 cm). Place side marker in the collimated exposure field.

kVp: 80   *Reference: 14th edition ATLAS p. 2:89.*

Manual Factors

Part Thickness (cm)	mA	kVp	Time	mAs	SID	Image Receptor Size	CR, DR Exposure Indicator	Grid	HF, 1Ø or 3Ø

AEC Factors

Part Thickness (cm)	mA	kVp	AEC Detector	mAs	Density Comp.	Image Receptor Size	CR, DR Exposure Indicator	Grid	HF, 1Ø or 3Ø

Notes: _____ Competency: _____/____/____

Instructor: _____

Cranium

Temporomandibular Articulations
Axiolateral oblique

Patient Position
• Position patient seated upright or semiprone.

Part Position
• Center a point ½ inch (1.3 cm) anterior to EAM to IR.
• Rotate midsagittal plane 15 degrees toward IR.
• Adjust AML parallel to transverse axis of IR.
• Interpupillary line is perpendicular to IR.
• After first exposure, do not permit patient to move. Change IR, and make second exposure with mouth fully open.

Respiration:
Suspend.

Central Ray
• Angle 15 degrees caudad, exiting temporomandibular joint closer to IR.
• Central ray enters about 1½ inches (3.8 cm) superior to upside EAM.

Collimation:
Adjust to extend from the outer canthus to the posterior edge of the auricle and from the midparietal region to the inferior edge of the auricle. The exposure field should be no larger than 5 × 5 inches (12.5 × 12.5 cm). Place side marker in the collimated exposure field.

kVp: 80

Reference: 14th edition ATLAS p. 2-93

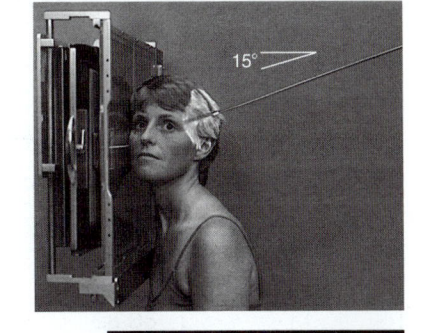

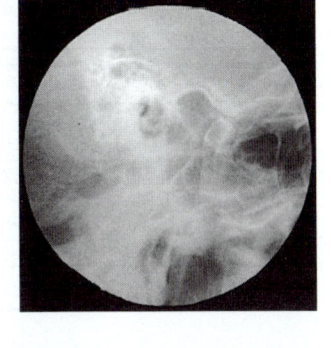

Manual Factors

Part Thickness (cm)	mA	kVp	Time	mAs	SID	Image Receptor Size	CR, DR Exposure Indicator	Grid	HF, 1Ø or 3Ø

AEC Factors

Part Thickness (cm)	mA	kVp	AEC Detector	mAs	Density Comp.	Image Receptor Size	CR, DR Exposure Indicator	Grid	HF, 1Ø or 3Ø

Notes: _____ Competency: ____/____/____

Instructor: _____

Cranium

Paranasal Sinuses
Lateral

Patient Position
• Position patient seated upright.

Part Position
• Adjust head to true lateral position.
• Midsagittal plane is parallel to (and interpupillary line is perpendicular to) IR.
• Adjust IOML horizontal and parallel to transverse axis of IR.

Respiration:
Suspend.

Central Ray
• Horizontal and perpendicular, entering ½ to 1 inch (1.3 to 2.5 cm) posterior to outer canthus.
• Center IR to central ray.

Collimation:
Adjust to extend ½ to 1 inch (1.3 to 2.5 cm) beyond the tip of the nose, superiorly to 3 inches above the nasion, inferiorly to the occlusal plane, and posteriorly to the auricle. The exposure field should be no larger than 8 × 10 inches (18 × 24 cm). Place side marker in the collimated exposure field.

kVp: 85

Reference: 14th edition ATLAS p. 2-98

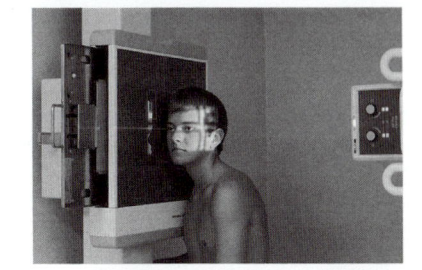

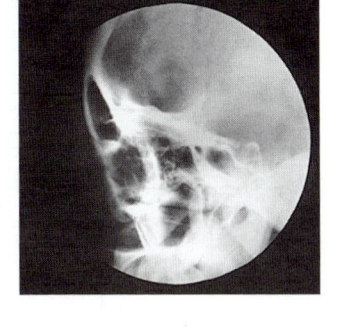

Manual Factors

Part Thickness (cm)	mA	kVp	Time	mAs	SID	Image Receptor Size	CR, DR Exposure Indicator	Grid	HF, 1Ø or 3Ø

AEC Factors

Part Thickness (cm)	mA	kVp	AEC Detector	mAs	Density Comp.	Image Receptor Size	CR, DR Exposure Indicator	Grid	HF, 1Ø or 3Ø

Notes: _____ Competency: _____/____/____

_____ Instructor: _____

Cranium

Frontal and Anterior Ethmoidal Sinuses
PA axial   CALDWELL METHOD

Patient Position
• Position patient seated upright.

Part Position
• Tilt vertical grid device down 15 degrees.
• Have patient rest head on forehead and nose.
• Position midsagittal plane perpendicular to midline of IR.
• OML is perpendicular to IR.
• This positioning places OML 15 degrees from horizontal central ray.

Respiration:
Suspend.

Central Ray
• Horizontal to center of IR, exiting nasion.

NOTE: If grid device cannot be tilted, place a radiolucent sponge between forehead and grid so that OML remains 15 degrees from horizontal x-ray beam.

Collimation:
Adjust to extend 1 inch (2.5 cm) beyond the lateral skin shadows, superiorly to include just the shadow of the top of the head, and inferiorly to the occlusal plane. The exposure field should be no larger than 8 × 10 inches (18 × 24 cm). Place side marker in the collimated exposure field.

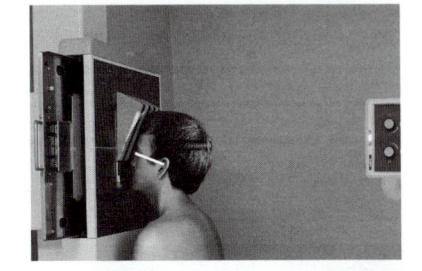

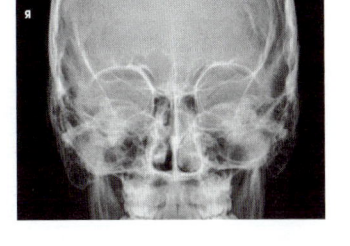

kVp: 85

Reference: 14th edition ATLAS p. 2:100

Manual Factors									
Part Thickness (cm)	mA	kVp	Time	mAs	SID	Image Receptor Size	CR, DR Exposure Indicator	Grid	HF, 1Ø or 3Ø

AEC Factors									
Part Thickness (cm)	mA	kVp	AEC Detector	mAs	Density Comp.	Image Receptor Size	CR, DR Exposure Indicator	Grid	HF, 1Ø or 3Ø

Notes: _____ Competency: ____/____/____

Instructor: _____

Cranium

Maxillary Sinuses
Parietoacanthial **WATERS METHOD**

Patient Position
• Position patient seated upright.

Part Position
• Center and adjust midsagittal plane perpendicular to IR, and have patient rest head on extended chin.
• Adjust OML to form 37-degree angle to IR. Mentomeatal line is approximately perpendicular to IR.
• Center IR to acanthion.
• *Open mouth option:* Have patient fully open mouth to show the sphenoid and maxillary sinuses.

Respiration:
Suspend.

Central Ray
• Horizontal and perpendicular to IR, exiting acanthion

Collimation:
Adjust to extend 1 inch (2.5 cm) beyond the lateral skin shadows, superiorly to include just the shadow of the top of the head, and inferiorly to the occlusal plane. The exposure field should be no larger than 8 × 10 inches (18 × 24 cm). Place side marker in the collimated exposure field.

kVp: 85

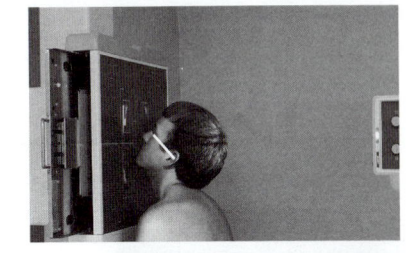
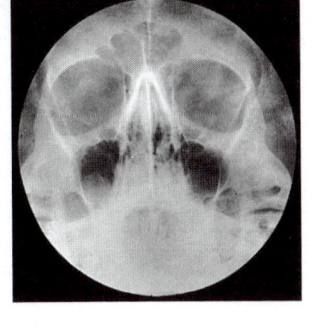

Manual Factors

Part Thickness (cm)	mA	kVp	Time	mAs	SID	Image Receptor Size	CR, DR Exposure Indicator	Grid	HF, 1Ø or 3Ø

AEC Factors

Part Thickness (cm)	mA	kVp	AEC Detector	mAs	Density Comp.	Image Receptor Size	CR, DR Exposure Indicator	Grid	HF, 1Ø or 3Ø

Notes: _____ Competency: ____/____/____

_____ Instructor: _____

Cranium

Ethmoidal and Sphenoidal Sinuses
Submentovertical

Patient Position
- Position patient seated upright at head unit.

Part Position
- Extend head, and have patient rest it on vertex.
- Center and adjust midsagittal plane perpendicular to IR.
- Adjust IOML parallel to IR.

Respiration:
Suspend.

Central Ray
- Horizontal and perpendicular to IOML.
- Central ray enters approximately ¾ inch (1.9 cm) anterior to level of EAM.

Collimation:
Adjust to extend ½ to 1 inch (1.3 to 2.5 cm) beyond the tip of the nose and on the lateral sides. The exposure field should be no larger than 8 × 10 inches (18 × 24 cm). Place side marker in the collimated exposure field.

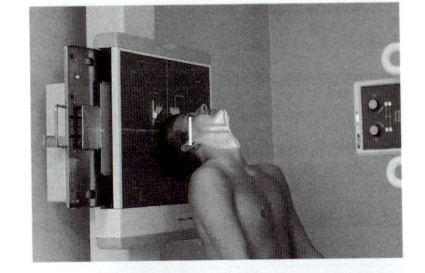

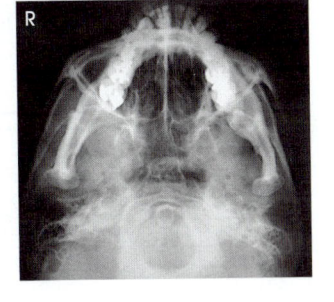

kVp: 85

Reference: 14th edition ATLAS p. 2:106.

Manual Factors

Part Thickness (cm)	mA	kVp	Time	mAs	SID	Image Receptor Size	CR, DR Exposure Indicator	Grid	HF, 1Ø or 3Ø

AEC Factors

Part Thickness (cm)	mA	kVp	AEC Detector	mAs	Density Comp.	Image Receptor Size	CR, DR Exposure Indicator	Grid	HF, 1Ø or 3Ø

Notes: _____ Competency: ____/____/____

Instructor: _____

Cranium

Chest:
AP, 320
AP or PA (right or left lateral decubitus), 322
Abdomen:
AP, 324
AP or PA (left lateral decubitus), 326

Pelvis:
AP, 328
Femur:
AP, 330
Lateral (dorsal decubitus), 332
Cervical Spine:
Lateral (right or left dorsal decubitus), 334

Chest and Abdomen: Neonate:
AP, 336
Lateral (right or left dorsal decubitus), 338

Mobile Radiography

Chest
AP

Patient Position
- Position patient upright or to greatest angle tolerated.
- Position critically ill or injured patients supine.

Part Position
- Center midsagittal plane to IR.
- Position IR under patient with top about 2 inches (5 cm) above relaxed shoulders.
- Internally rotate patient's arms to prevent scapular superimposition of lung field, if not contraindicated.
- Ensure that patient's upper torso is not rotated.
- Shield gonads

Respiration:
Inspiration.

Central Ray
- Perpendicular to center of IR.

Collimation:
Adjust to 14 × 17 inches (35 × 43 cm). Place side marker in the collimated exposure field.

kVp: 90 (40" SID, non-grid), 105 (40" grid)

Reference: 14th edition ATLAS p. 3:10.

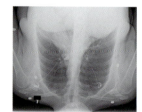

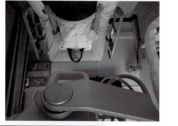

Manual Factors									
Part Thickness (cm)	mA	kVp	Time	mAs	SID	Image Receptor Size	CR, DR Exposure Indicator	Grid	HF, 1Ø or 3Ø

Notes: _____ Competency: _____/___/___

_____ Instructor: _____

Mobile Radiography

Chest
AP or PA (right or left lateral decubitus)

Patient Position
- Position patient in lateral recumbent position.
- Place firm support under patient to elevate body 2 to 3 inches (5 to 7.5 cm).
- Raise both arms up and away from chest region.
- Ensure that patient cannot fall out of bed.

Part Position
- Perform AP projection whenever possible.
- Adjust patient to ensure true lateral position.
- Place IR behind patient and below support.
- Adjust grid so that it extends 2 inches (5 cm) above shoulders.
- Shield gonads.

Respiration:
Inspiration.

Central Ray
- Horizontal and perpendicular to center of IR.

Collimation:
Adjust to 14 × 17 inches (35 × 43 cm). Place side marker in the collimated exposure field.

kVp: 105 (40″ grid)

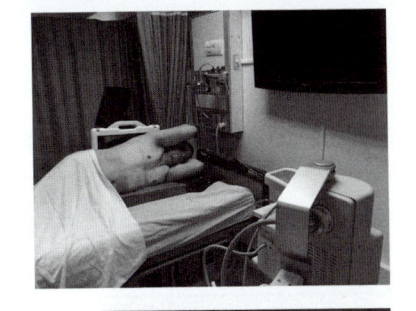

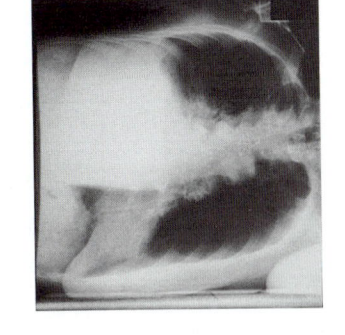

Manual Factors

Part Thickness (cm)	mA	kVp	Time	mAs	SID	Image Receptor Size	CR, DR Exposure Indicator	Grid	HF, 1Ø or 3Ø

Notes: _____ Competency: _____/_____/_____

_____ Instructor: _____

Mobile Radiography

Abdomen
AP

Patient Position
• Position patient supine using horizontal bed placement.

Part Position
• Position grid under patient.
• Keep grid from tipping side to side by placing it in center of bed and stabilizing with blankets if necessary.
• Center midsagittal plane to grid.
• If emphasis is on upper abdomen, center grid 2 inches (5 cm) above iliac crests or high enough to include diaphragm.
• Shield gonads.

Respiration:
Suspended.

Central Ray
• Perpendicular to center of grid at level of iliac crests.

Collimation:
Adjust to 14 × 17 inches (35 × 43 cm). Place side marker in the collimated exposure field.

kVp: 85   *Reference: 14th edition ATLAS p. 3:14.*

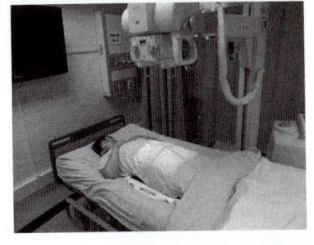

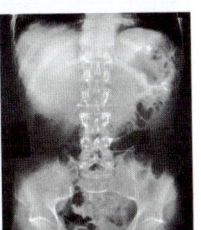

Manual Factors									
Part Thickness (cm)	mA	kVp	Time	mAs	SID	Image Receptor Size	CR, DR Exposure Indicator	Grid	HF, 1Ø or 3Ø

Notes: _____ Competency: _____/___/___

_____ Instructor: _____

Mobile Radiography

Abdomen
AP or PA (left lateral decubitus)

Patient Position
- Place patient in left lateral recumbent position.
- If necessary, place firm support under patient to elevate body.
- Ensure that patient cannot fall out of bed.

Part Position
- Adjust patient to ensure true lateral position.
- Place grid vertically in front of patient for PA or behind patient for AP. Support grid to prevent grid cutoff.
- Position grid so that its center is 2 inches (5 cm) above iliac crests to ensure that diaphragm is included.
- Shield gonads.

Respiration:
Suspended.

Central Ray
- Horizontal and perpendicular to center of grid.

Collimation:
Adjust to 14 × 17 inches (35 × 43 cm). Place side marker in the collimated exposure field.

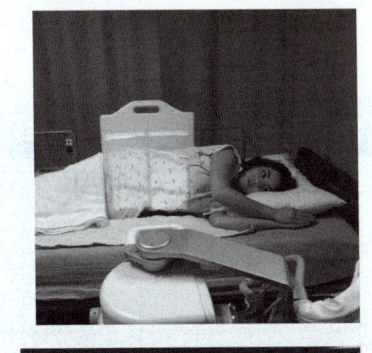

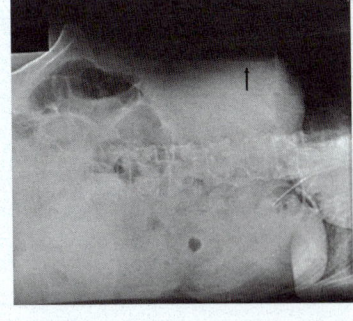

kVp: 85

Reference: 14th edition ATLAS p. 3-16

Manual Factors									
Part Thickness (cm)	mA	kVp	Time	mAs	SID	Image Receptor Size	CR, DR Exposure Indicator	Grid	HF, 1Ø or 3Ø

Notes: _____ Competency: _____/_____/_____

_____ Instructor: _____

Mobile Radiography

Pelvis
AP

Patient Position
• Position patient supine.

Part Position
• Position grid under pelvis so that center is midway between ASIS and pubic symphysis (about 2 inches [5 cm] inferior to ASIS).
• Center midsagittal plane to midline of grid. Pelvis should not be rotated.
• Rotate patient's legs medially 15 degrees when not contraindicated.

Respiration:
Suspend.

Central Ray
• Perpendicular to midpoint of grid. Central ray should enter patient 2 inches (5 cm) above pubic symphysis and 2 inches (5 cm) below ASIS.

Collimation:
Adjust to 14 × 17 inches (35 × 43 cm). Place side marker in the collimated exposure field.

kVp: 85

Reference: 14th edition ATLAS p. 3:18.

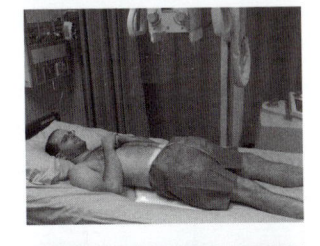
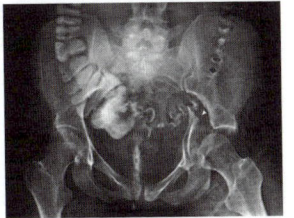

Manual Factors									
Part Thickness (cm)	mA	kVp	Time	mAs	SID	Image Receptor Size	CR, DR Exposure Indicator	Grid	HF, 1Ø or 3Ø

Notes: _____ Competency: ____/____/____

_____ Instructor: _____

Mobile Radiography

Femur
AP

Patient Position
- Position patient supine.

Part Position
- *Cautiously* place grid lengthwise under patient's femur, with distal edge of grid low enough to include fracture site and knee joint.
- Elevate grid with towels under each side to ensure proper grid alignment with x-ray tube.
- Center grid to midline of femur.
- Shield gonads.

Respiration:
Suspend.

Central Ray
- Perpendicular to long axis of femur; center to grid.
- Ensure that central ray and grid are aligned to prevent grid cutoff.

Collimation:
Adjust to 1 inch (2.5 cm) on sides of shadow of femur and 17 inches (43 cm) in length. Place side marker in the collimated exposure field.

kVp: 85

Reference: 14th edition ATLAS p. 3:20.

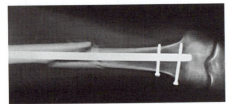

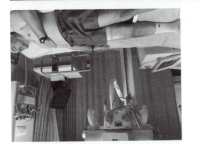

Manual Factors									
Part Thickness (cm)	mA	kVp	Time	mAs	SID	Image Receptor Size	CR, DR Exposure Indicator	Grid	HF, 1Ø or 3Ø

Notes: _____ Competency: ____/____/____

_____ Instructor: _____

Mobile Radiography

Femur
Lateral (dorsal decubitus)

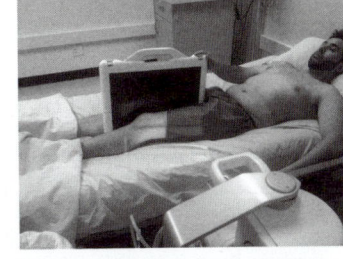

Patient Position
• Position patient supine.

Part Position
• Determine whether mediolateral or lateromedial projection is to be performed.
• Place grid in vertical position next to lateral aspect of femur.
• Place distal edge of grid low enough to include knee joint.
• Stabilize grid firmly in position (patient may hold).
• Support and elevate unaffected leg.
• Ensure that grid is placed perpendicular to epicondylar plane.

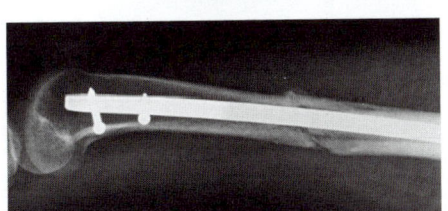

Respiration:
Suspend.

Central Ray
• Perpendicular to long axis of femur; center to grid.

Collimation:
Adjust to 1 inch (2.5 cm) on sides of shadow of femur and 17 inches (43 cm) in length. Place side marker in the collimated exposure field.

kVp: 85

Reference: 14th edition ATLAS p. 3:22.

Manual Factors

Part Thickness (cm)	mA	kVp	Time	mAs	SID	Image Receptor Size	CR, DR Exposure Indicator	Grid	HF, 1Ø or 3Ø

Notes: _____ Competency: _____/___/___

_____ Instructor: _____

Mobile Radiography

Cervical Spine
Lateral (right or left dorsal decubitus)

Patient Position
- Position patient supine with arms extended along sides of body.
- *Do not remove cervical collar without consent of physician.*

Part Position
- Ensure that upper torso and head are not rotated.
- Place grid lengthwise on right or left side, parallel to neck.
- Place top of grid 1 to 2 inches (2.5 to 5 cm) above EAM.
- Immobilize grid in vertical position.
- Have patient relax shoulders and reach for feet if possible.

Respiration:
Full expiration.

Central Ray
- Horizontal and perpendicular to center of grid.
- Use SID of 60 to 72 inches (158 to 183 cm).

Collimation:
Adjust to 10 × 12 inches (24 × 30 cm). Place side marker in the collimated exposure field.

kVp: 85

Reference: 14th edition ATLAS p. 3:24.

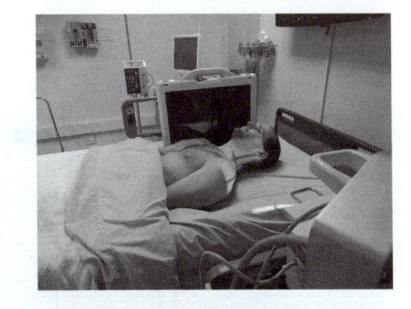

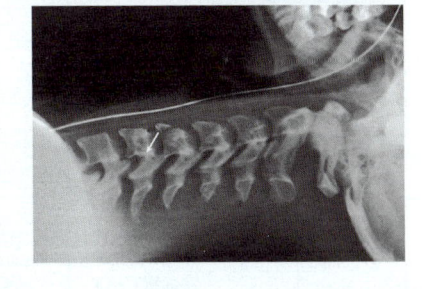

Manual Factors

Part Thickness (cm)	mA	kVp	Time	mAs	SID	Image Receptor Size	CR, DR Exposure Indicator	Grid	HF, 1Ø or 3Ø

Notes: _____ Competency: _____/____/____

_____ Instructor: _____

Mobile Radiography

Chest and Abdomen: Neonate
AP

Patient Position
• Position patient supine in center of IR. If IR is directly under infant, cover IR with soft, warm blanket.

Part Position
• *Carefully* position x-ray tube over infant.
• Ensure that chest and abdomen are not rotated.
• Move infant's arms away from body, and bring legs down and away from abdomen.
• Leave infant's head rotated.
• Shield gonads.

Respiration:
Inspiration.

Central Ray
• Perpendicular to midpoint of chest and abdomen.

Collimation:
Adjust to 1 inch (2.5 cm) on all sides of chest and abdomen. Place side marker in the collimated exposure field.

kVp: 64

Reference: 14th edition ATLAS p. 3:26.

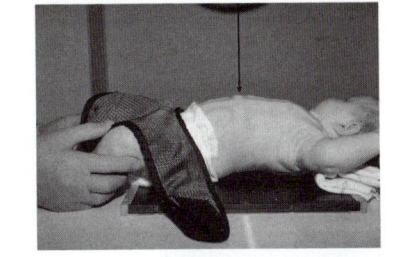

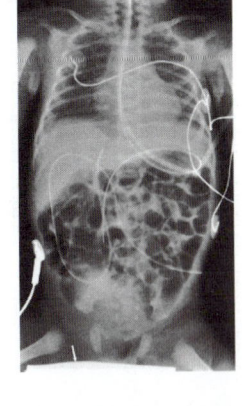

Manual Factors									
Part Thickness (cm)	mA	kVp	Time	mAs	SID	Image Receptor Size	CR, DR Exposure Indicator	Grid	HF, 1Ø or 3Ø

Notes: _____ Competency: _____/___/___

_____ Instructor: _____

Mobile Radiography

Chest and Abdomen: Neonate
Lateral (right or left dorsal decubitus)

Patient Position
- *Carefully* place x-ray tube to side of bassinet.
- Position infant supine on radiolucent block covered with soft, warm blanket.

Part Position
- Ensure that infant's chest and abdomen are centered to IR and not rotated.
- Move infant's arms above head.
- Place IR lengthwise and vertical beside infant, then immobilize IR.
- Leave infant's head rotated.
- Shield gonads.

Respiration:
Inspiration.

Central Ray
- Horizontal and perpendicular to midpoint of chest and abdomen along midcoronal plane.

Collimation:
Adjust to length of chest and abdomen and 1 inch (2.5 cm) above abdomen. Place side marker in the collimated exposure field.

kVp: 72

Reference: 14th edition ATLAS p. 2:20

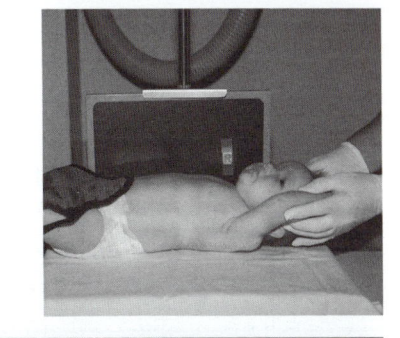

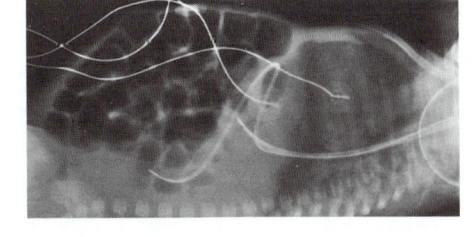

Manual Factors									
Part Thickness (cm)	mA	kVp	Time	mAs	SID	Image Receptor Size	CR, DR Exposure Indicator	Grid	HF, 1Ø or 3Ø

Notes: _____ Competency: ____/____/____

_____ Instructor: _____

Mobile Radiography

SID Conversion, 342

Grid Conversion Factors, 344

Appendices

SID Conversion

When SID* is changed, mAs must be changed to compensate for differences in radiation intensity. To use, locate the original SID on the left-hand vertical column of the accompanying chart. Read across the chart to the column under the desired (new) SID. Multiply the original mAs by the conversion factor (from the box) to obtain the new mAs (e.g., using 15 mAs at 40 inches changing to 60 inches, 15 mAs × 2.25 = 33.75 mAs at 60 inches SID).

*Source-to-image–receptor distance.

Desired SID

Original SID \ Distance	36"	40"	44"	48"	52"	56"	60"	64"	68"	72"
36"	1.0	1.23	1.5	1.78	2.09	2.42	2.78	3.16	3.57	4.0
40"	0.81	1.0	1.21	1.44	1.69	1.96	2.25	2.56	2.89	3.24
44"	0.67	0.83	1.0	1.19	1.4	1.62	1.86	2.12	2.39	2.68
48"	0.56	0.69	0.84	1.0	1.17	1.36	1.56	1.78	2.01	2.25
52"	0.48	0.59	0.72	0.85	1.0	1.16	1.33	1.51	1.71	1.92
56"	0.41	0.51	0.62	0.73	0.86	1.0	1.15	1.31	1.47	1.65
60"	0.36	0.44	0.54	0.64	0.75	0.87	1.0	1.14	1.28	1.44
64"	0.32	0.39	0.47	0.56	0.66	0.77	0.88	1.0	1.13	1.27
68"	0.28	0.35	0.42	0.5	0.58	0.68	0.78	0.89	1.0	1.12
72"	0.25	0.31	0.37	0.44	0.52	0.6	0.69	0.79	0.89	1.0

Appendices

Grid Conversion Factors

When converting from one grid ratio to another, use the following formula:

$$\frac{mAs\ 1}{mAs\ 2} = \frac{GCF\ 1}{GCF\ 2}$$

Where:
- $mAs\ 1$ = original mAs
- $mAs\ 2$ = new mAs
- $GCF\ 1$ = original grid conversion factor
- $GCF\ 2$ = new grid conversion factor

Grid Ratio	60 kVp	85 kVp	110 kVp
No grid	1	1	1
5:1	3	3	3
8:1	3.75	4	4.25
12:1	4.75	5.5	6.25
16:1	5:75	6:75	8

Adapted from Characteristics and applications of x-ray grids, *Cincinnati, 1992, Liebel-Flarsheim division of Sybron Corporation. Approximate values based on clinical tests of pelvis and skull.*

Closely collimated radiographs require an increase in exposure to maintain a comparable density to compensate for the decrease in scatter radiation reaching the image receptor. Approximate changes in exposure are suggested as follows:

Collimating from	To	Increase mAs by
14 × 17 inches (35 × 43 cm)	10 × 12 inches (24 × 30 cm)	25%
14 × 17 inches (35 × 43 cm)	8 × 10 inches (18 × 24 cm)	40%
14 × 17 inches (35 × 43 cm)	5 × 7 inches (13 × 18 cm)	60%

Orthopedic Cast Technique

Radiographic techniques generally need to be increased to penetrate orthopedic casts. The amount of exposure increase depends on the thickness of the cast, cast material, and x-ray energy. The following techniques are suggested as guidelines for initial adjustment:

	Increase Exposure by
For dry plaster cast	2 × mAs, or + 10 kVp
For wet plaster cast	3 × mAs, or 2 + mAs and +10 kVp
For fiberglass cast	+ 5 to +8 kVp

Notes:

Notes

Notes

Notes

Notes

Notes

Notes

Notes

Notes

Notes